Dictionary of Syndromes and Inherited Disorders

Dictionary of Syndromes and Inherited Disorders

3rd Edition

Patricia Gilbert

CHICAGO • LONDON

FITZROY DEARBORN PUBLISHERS
919 North Michigan Avenue
Chicago, Illinois 60611
USA

or

FITZROY DEARBORN PUBLISHERS
310 Regent Street
London W1R 5AJ
England

British Library and Library of Congress Cataloguing in Publication Data are available.

ISBN 1-57958-226-5

First published in the USA 2000
This edition first published in the UK 2000

Contents

Foreword

More often than not, my heart sinks when I know I am to see a family with a child who has a "syndrome." It sinks because it is highly likely that I will not understand the cause of the syndrome, because there may be no specific treatment, because the outlook (particularly in newly described syndromes) may be unknown, and, most importantly, because the parents will ask me sensible and pertinent questions that I cannot answer. Only if I have special expertise in the disorder, or group of disorders, will I be able to help the child as I would wish. Clearly, I cannot have expertise in, or knowledge of, even a fraction of the more than 2,000 syndromes now described.

My difficulties are, I am sure, shared to a greater or lesser extent by all who may be involved in counseling, or caring for, those handicapped by a syndrome. Many who will be responsible for providing for the child's needs, and to whom the parents may turn, may not even have any background medical knowledge. This book, written simply and concisely and in nontechnical language, gives just the sort of information needed. It will be a boon to those working in child health in the community, in social services, and in schools.

To cover more than a small selection of the known syndromes is clearly impracticable, and to be always up-to-date with the latest "discovery" in such a rapidly moving field is impossible. Dr. Gilbert, with her extensive experience, has chosen wisely, and much of the practical information that she gives will not become out of date. Patients, parents, and professionals will have reason to be grateful to her for having compiled this compendium on a difficult and important topic.

Professor Dame June Lloyd

Preface

Syndromes are part of everyday diagnosis today. The number described seems to increase weekly. Hitherto, few were known or documented accurately. Just what are these conditions so labeled?

The Oxford English Dictionary defines a *syndrome* as "a concurrence of several symptoms in a disease; a set of such concurrent symptoms." Put in simpler terms, a syndrome can be described as a specific collection of signs and symptoms that, when put together, form a recognizable pattern that can be seen to be repeated in another individual.

There are now many thousands of these syndromes recorded. Some are incredibly rare, others uncommon, while others are relatively frequently seen. For example, in the latter group is Down syndrome—well-known to most people—with a general incidence of 1 in approximately every 800 births. Examples of the rarer syndromes are Hunter and Hurler syndromes. Both of these syndromes are only found in 1 child in 100,000. Few doctors, nurses, teachers, or social workers (unless their work happened to be with handicapped children or adults) will have seen more than a handful of such syndromes. Nevertheless, as the number of classified syndromes increases, many of these professionals could well be seeing several people with a specific syndrome during their working life.

At some time during the lives of people who have a definable syndrome, and most commonly in childhood, help in some form, be it medical, nursing, social, or educational, will be needed. In the early days, parents will need support, advice, and counseling in order to come to terms with their child's disability, as well as guidance concerning practical aspects of care. Later in the child's life, social workers and educators become involved. All these professionals need accurate knowledge of each specific syndrome if they are to be fully effective in their support of families.

In this book, a small number of the known syndromes, alphabetically listed, are described. Each section gives guidelines on the practical aspects of help that can be given. Any one of the disciplines of medicine, nursing, social work, or education may be involved, but in many cases, all four disciplines will have a part to play. Many of the syndromes have self-help groups; these groups have frequently been set up by parents who themselves have a child with the specific disorder. Contact points for these self-help groups are to be found at the end of each appropriate section. The effects of a handicapping condition on the individual, the family, and society in general are discussed separately. Comprehensive cross-indexing is included to help the reader toward the correct syndrome. For instance, all syndromes having short stature as a characteristic are listed together in the index, as are those syndromes in which a lazy eye might be a factor.

It is hoped that this book will prove to be of value to all professionals who are concerned with the care of handicapped children. It has been difficult to limit the number of syndromes described to a manageable minimum. The main criteria that have been involved in this choice are two-fold. First, the syndrome must result in long-term, and in many cases lifelong, mental and/or physical problems of one kind or another. Second, help must be available that can alleviate some of the problems and improve the quality of life. The author will be pleased to receive comments and suggestions as to possible further inclusions at a later date.

Finally, my thanks are due to all the many children with a syndrome, and their parents, with whom I have had the privilege to work over the years.

Preface to the Third Edition

Twenty extra syndromes have been added to this third edition, bringing the total described to 100. A number of the added syndromes have been specifically requested by readers, to whom I give my thanks.

The same criteria for inclusion have been applied as in the original text. The entire text has been extensively revised in an endeavor to keep up with the rapidly expanding knowledge associated with genetic conditions.

The glossary has also been extended to include a greater number of more common medical terms. It is hoped that this section will prove helpful to the general readership.

Acknowledgments

My thanks are due to a number of people who have given encouragement and help with the writing of this book. In particular, Dr. Terry Billington has given unstintingly of her time and expertise in reading the manuscript. Without her medical and physical therapy skills, much would have been lost. Dr. Peter Farndon also has found time in his exceedingly busy life to give advice on the genetics references, and I am in his debt for his assistance. It must be emphasized, however, that any errors in the text are entirely my own.

Much gratitude is also felt to Professor June Lloyd for writing the foreword to the first edition, and I would like to thank her again for her kind words and sentiments.

Rosemary Morris and Tony Wayte have been unstinting in their enthusiasm and encouragement. Without their ready availability and professional expertise, my task would have been more difficult.

Finally, my thanks are again given to my husband, who has continued to guide me successfully through the minefields of word-processing with patience and cheerfulness throughout the various editions of this book.

The Effects of Handicap

Our genetic inheritance colors all our life. The medical conditions passed down the family line will affect our daily lives as surely as do our height, the color of our skin, and our potential for low or high ability. And when a syndrome, or specifically inherited condition, is part of our family tree, its effects can be very great indeed. Our family, our friends, and the wider society in which we live will all be affected by our genetic inheritance to a greater or lesser degree. These effects will not cease when childhood is outgrown. The whole of our adult life will be altered, for better or worse.

Between 15 and 20% of adults suffer from some chronic condition that has a bearing on some, or all, of their daily living. Some of these problems are due, of course, to reasons other than inherited disease. Infection and environmental factors all play their part, but it is thought that some 16% of all babies born alive have some defect, many of which are small and insignificant, at birth. About half of these babies will have a condition that will give rise to functional problems of one kind or another throughout their lives. Therefore, this aspect of life will have an impact on very many people, whether directly in a day-to-day manner, in the work environment, or merely in a chance encounter.

Obviously, the greatest effect of an inherited disease will be felt by each individual having the specific condition. Every baby has the same basic needs of warmth, food, love, and a sense of belonging. All but the most unfortunate babies will have the first two of these necessities met (although genetic inheritance may cause difficulties of adequate nutrition in some babies, quite apart from economic factors). It is love and, later, a sense of belonging that some severely disabled babies can lack. Parents, who have waited for nine long months for the arrival of a perfect baby, can be distraught at the sight of a handicapped newcomer. Those caring for the parents and baby will need to handle the situation carefully and sensitively. The majority of parents, under these circumstances, will accept their baby with love, but a few may take time to come to terms with the unexpected problems facing them. Fortunately, relatively few parents completely reject their handicapped child.

Later in the child's life, problems of acceptance can also occur. Such problems can especially arise when the child has an inherited disorder needing much daily—and possibly nightly—care. Parents can become completely exhausted by the unremitting and inevitable demands of their handicapped child. Child abuse, in any one of a number of guises, may

1

occur, and it must be remembered as a possibility under these circumstances. Doctors, nurses and social workers, and also teachers when schooldays are reached, should all be aware of the strain under which the parents of a handicapped child are living. Help, be it practical, financial, or psychological, should be made available before the burdens become intolerable.

A further basic need of childhood, and indeed throughout life, is the need to be able to continue to learn. Children with handicaps can often miss out on this vital aspect of normal living. To avoid this problem, the precise diagnosis of his/her condition must be made initially. Following diagnosis, assessment of the effects of the syndrome on various functions—vision, hearing, and mobility, to mention just a few—will be needed. Only then can a specific program of learning, at whatever basic level, be organized. It is important that the exact nature of the disability is diagnosed early. Vital stages of learning can be missed if a child's handicap is not discovered quickly. For example, a baby born with a profound hearing loss will rarely, if ever, be able to speak unless the hearing problem is recognized and appropriate treatment and training given. Similarly, legally blind children may have a little residual vision, but their sight will be too limited for the learning process to proceed normally. Therefore, suitable educational facilities for learning by methods involving touch must be organized. These are but two examples of the ways in which an inherited disease, or a syndrome, can affect an individual's capacity to meet the basic needs of life.

Parents, too, should be carefully advised on what activities are most suitable for the developmental age of their child. In many syndromes that have a degree of mental retardation as part of the symptomatology, chronological age is no guide to the stage of development the child has reached. For example, a child with Down syndrome is frequently behind his/her contemporaries in many aspects of mobility. His/her walking will be delayed due to the almost universal hypotonia found in children with Down syndrome. Therefore, it is inadvisable for parents to buy toys that are designed for children with early onset of this particular skill. Later, as the child with this handicap falls further behind his/her peers, toys and activities will need to be geared to his/her mental abilities rather than to his/her physical age.

A further aspect of life with an inherited handicapping condition is the possible need for frequent hospital admissions. Hospitalization can have two major effects on the life of the individual child. The child will be away from his/her immediate family and friends for, sometimes long, periods of time. These absences can loosen the ties of everyday involvement with work and play. For the older child, when school days are a reality, lessons are also missed unless there can be close cooperation among school, home, and hospital. During an acute bout of illness, school work obviously cannot be considered, but during convalescence, time can usefully, and happily, be spent catching up with class work. This observation especially applies to children with such conditions as cystic fibrosis and osteogenesis imperfecta, for example. For children with these two conditions (and many others), hospitalization can be a recurrent necessity. All efforts to maintain contact with family and friends should be made.

Finally, when considering the effects of handicap on a particular child, we must never forget to appreciate her or him as an individual. It is all too easy to talk down to a child in a wheelchair who has perhaps an added speech or hearing problem. It is important, especially as the teenage years are reached, that these young people should be involved in decisions as to their future, if at all possible. Deciding whether later schooling should be in a special school or in a mainstream facility with added resources is an issue that involves the child as much as—or perhaps more than—the parents. Choices must be worked out with the child's comments and feelings an important part of the discussion.

Careers, if applicable, must also be a decision made jointly by child, parent, and adviser. Some handicaps will, of course, prevent a person from pursuing any of the more active careers, but many conditions do allow the individual to work alongside peers who have no such disability. Particular activities may require extra considerations, such as ramps for those people with a mobility problem or extra light for persons with poor vision, for instance. Possible complications must be evaluated carefully, but the wishes of the young person should be an important part of the final decision.

To summarize how parents and professionals involved in the care of a child with a handicap can make life as normal as possible:

- All efforts should be made to learn as much as possible about the condition from which the child is suffering. Knowing which difficulties the child has to overcome is half the process of to helping him/her to cope with his/her disability. For instance, try to see what life is really like with only central (or "tunnel") vision by cutting off the range of side vision with a hood. Crossing the road safely becomes twice as difficult, and people coming up quietly behind you can be fairly frightening. Or, tie one arm behind you to find out just how difficult it is to perform many everyday activities with only one functioning arm. These experiments, of course, are gross examples, and ones easily replicated. It is much more difficult to understand the problems encountered by children with poor cognitive abilities, whose surroundings make little sense to them. However, such an understanding is just what care givers should try to acquire, so that the best possible help can be given.

■ Find out how the specific condition may progress. What will the child be doing and feeling when, say, five years have passed? Syndromes and other inherited disorders vary greatly in the way they progress—some may reach a plateau and stay there for many years, while others, regrettably, progress rapidly. Many syndromes have self-help groups, often started by parents who themselves have a child with the particular condition. Through such organizations, other persons affected by the same, or similar, condition can correspond or even meet to compare notes on various problems and how best to overcome them. Much information can be gained on practical aspects of daily living and benefits obtainable, as well as friendship, from such sources.

■ All parents have ambitions for their children. When their son or daughter has been found to have a specific handicapping condition, these ambitions will have to be substantially altered. Sometimes, with a severely affected child, the outlook for life itself is limited. With yet other serious disorders, parents will be forced to accept that only the most minimal of self-help skills will ever be attained. This realization can be devastatingly difficult for even the most mature and sympathetic parent, but from the child's point of view, it is of immense significance that the adjustment is made so realistic boundaries can then be set. Here again, sympathetic help from others in similar circumstances can be of enormous value.

■ Children who need hospitalization can be prepared for these events. Finding out about admission procedures, what clothing to take, toys allowed, and many other day-to-day events can do much to alleviate the fear of the unknown. A positive attitude from the parents themselves concerning the outcome of the perhaps extended and painful procedures will serve to minimize the upsets of admission to the hospital. While the child is actually in the hospital, regular visits with small gifts, photographs of family, and day-to-day updates about home news can do much to negate feelings of isolation.

Close liaison with medical and nursing staff regarding the type and length of proposed treatments can help parents explain to their child what is likely to happen within the next day or two. Nowadays, most hospitals welcome parents to be with their child when at all possible during treatment. For example, parents are able to be with their child immediately before anesthesia, and also to be at their child's side when he/she re-awakens.

- Diets necessary to the well-being of the handicapped child can be at times unpalatable and different from the foods the child's friends are eating. Food can be made as palatable as possible, and explanations can be given to friends about the necessity for any restrictions.
- Finally, it must be remembered that children who have a syndrome are much more likely to have some behavioral disorder than their peers. Such behavioral problems are in addition to the effects of the disorder itself. If parents are warned of this possibility and are counseled as to how best to avoid these problems, the incidence of outbursts will be reduced to a minimum.

These then are some of the aspects an inherited disorder can have on the individual child. But what about the parents, who, instead of their hoped-for perfect son or daughter, are faced with a baby who, in addition to looking "different," has the prospect of needing special, continuing care for many years?

The immediate reaction to the birth of an obviously handicapped baby is one of shock and disbelief. Both parents will need sensitive, and ongoing, sympathy and counseling if they are both to accept their baby as he/she is. They must be allowed to grieve, for the birth of handicapped child is surely almost as much a bereavement as is a stillbirth. All the hopes and aspirations for a perfect, healthy baby are dashed in one brief moment. Parents need time and space to come to terms with their loss. All the usual grief reactions will be there—disbelief, anger, guilt, depression, and finally acceptance. These stages will, of course, vary from person to person. Some mothers will find it easy to love and care for their babies, while others will feel more traumatized. The father, too, must not be forgotten. He may be very supportive, but he, as well, will need to work through his disappointment. Thankfully, the vast majority of parents come to terms with the outcome of the pregnancy and continue, often for many years, to love and care for their handicapped child. Later, as the child grows and possibly becomes more and more demanding of the parents' time and energies, their marriage may be put under severe strain. If there are other children, they can become resentful of all the attention paid to their handicapped brother or sister. These situations need much thought and sensitive counseling to resolve.

Perhaps an even greater shock occurs when the baby appears to be perfect at birth and then a genetic disorder begins to show itself in the first few months or years of life. For example, babies with Hunter syndrome are normal at birth, but they begin to deteriorate physically and mentally around 18 months to 2 years old. If diagnosis serves to confirm fears of an inherited disorder, parents will go through similar grief reactions as did other parents who have a child with a genetic disorder that was obvious at birth, such as Down syndrome or Apert syndrome (for example).

Genetic disorders can also generate a good deal of guilty feelings in the parents, who feel that it is their fault that their child has been born with the particular syndrome. Again, explanation of the ways of genetic inheritance can help to overcome some of these feelings.

The wider family, not to mention close friends (who may also be in the reproductive years themselves), will be affected by the birth, or subsequent development, of a handicapped child. Parents who have accurate knowledge of their baby's condition will be in a better position to answer queries as to what is wrong with their baby and how the condition will affect the life of the family in the future.

A handicapped child can bring families closer together in their support for the parents and the care of the child. Friends, too, will often rally round and give practical help and moral support. Occasionally, however, the opposite reaction occurs, and contact with parents and their baby ceases abruptly. With a handicapped child, one learns quickly who is a friend!

Life is never the same after the birth of any baby. With the birth of a handicapped baby, this change is increased a hundredfold. Hospital and clinic visits will need to be fitted into the daily routine; special treatments or foods may need to be given; or in-patient spells may be necessary. All of these adjustments come on top of caring for a physically and/or mentally handicapped child who is not developing along the same lines as other babies. No wonder parents became quite exhausted, particularly as normal sleep patterns in the baby may be difficult to establish. Help from a variety of agencies should be made available to parents who have a baby suffering under these, or similar, conditions.

Accurate **diagnosis** is one of the most important first steps in adjusting to a child's needs. Following the diagnosis, information can then be given as to what the future holds. Absorbing such information can take up much time, as parents will need to think about the implications for their future lives. During this time of adjustment, many potential day-to-day problems will occur to them. Therefore, it is necessary to emphasize once again that an important part of helping parents to come to terms with their baby's handicap is allowing time—maybe again and again—for discussion. Worries and fears need to be voiced so that explanations can be given, together with information on various agencies that can offer practical help.

Social workers will need to be involved with the family from the early days. Advice on help available, be it financial assistance or local chapters of support groups (for example), can do much to relieve the isolation felt by parents.

Self-help groups, a number of which have been formed over the past decade, can also provide much support. It is good to be able to write, meet with, or telephone a family that has a child with a similar syndrome. Day-to-day management of problems can be talked over informally. Many of these self-help groups provide useful material on the specific condition and can arrange meetings for members. Many of these self-help groups also organize fund-raising activities for research. These groups, together with social worker input, give valuable information regarding various items of equipment available for disabled living.

It is important that every handicapped child has his/her abilities, both physical and mental, **assessed** regularly on an ongoing basis. These assessments can be done at a hospital, at a clinic specializing in this purpose, or at the child's own doctor's office if that physician is particularly interested in such problems.

Genetic counseling, if the parents are contemplating a further pregnancy, is important after the birth of a handicapped child. The exact diagnosis of the handicapping condition will need to be known, and a family tree identifying any other similarly handicapped members will need to be created. Genetic counseling services are available at most university teaching hospitals. Any future pregnancy must be monitored carefully, with techniques such as ultrasound, chorionic villus sampling, and amniocentesis.

Finally, **bereavement counseling** may be necessary at a later date. Many children with specific handicapping conditions cannot look forward to a normal life span. In a number of syndromes, death can occur in the late teenage years or early 20s. Even though they have been led to expect this loss, the actual event is a shattering blow to parents. After a busy life caring for their handicapped child, the days suddenly seem long and empty. Feelings of relief are mixed with the inevitable feelings of sadness and loss. Such emotions can lead to an excess of the guilt normally felt after a death: "Perhaps there could have been more done for our child?" "Perhaps we were not as dedicated as we should have been?"

And most pertinent of all in a genetically acquired condition, "Was it our fault?" Parents will need much sympathetic support during the weeks and months following the death of a handicapped child.

All is not gloom, however, following the birth of a child with an inherited handicap. Families can be brought closer together in the care of their child. Pleasure can also result from helping with the everyday successes of life with a handicap. Many families will be certain that their quality of life is enhanced by their handicapped child with his/her own unique personality.

As our knowledge of the causes and effects of handicap increases, more help will be given to members of our society—all over the world.

Achondroplasia

ALTERNATIVE NAME

Chondro-dystrophy.

INCIDENCE

The incidence of achondroplasia is thought to be around 1 in every 25,000 births. The mode of inheritance would suggest this figure is variable, due to the inability to predict new mutations, which can also result in achondroplasia. Both sexes can be affected, and it is possible to diagnose achondroplasia at birth. A number of achondroplastic pregnancies are known to miscarry, or the baby dies in the early weeks of life, particularly if the birth has been premature.

HISTORY

There are quite a large number of conditions and syndromes in which short stature is a prominent feature. Achondroplasia is unique in that the limbs are short, while the trunk is of a normal size. This abnormality is obvious at birth, while the short stature of other conditions will only become obvious as the child matures.

Many achondroplastic men and women used to be the "small people" working in circuses. This work was the only occupation open to them until comparatively recently, when enlightenment regarding suitable careers became the societal norm. Achondroplasia is now no bar to many jobs and professions, including medicine and teaching.

CAUSATION

The mode of inheritance is twofold. Achondroplasia can be inherited as an autosomal dominant characteristic, or it can arise as a new mutation. It is thought that the latter mode of inheritance accounts for most of the babies born with achondroplasia. It has been suggested that advanced paternal age may be a factor, but this hypothesis has not been proved. The basic fault is that the epiphyseal plates of the limbs fail to produce adequate cartilage tissue. This process starts before birth.

CHARACTERISTICS

Short stature: This is of a very particular type. The arms and legs are short, while the trunk and head are of normal size. Specialist charts are currently being produced to monitor the growth of achondroplastic children. Due to the disproportion in the body configuration in an achondroplastic child, the usual charts will not give a true picture of whether or not the child is growing satisfactorily.

Head size appears out of proportion to the trunk. There are a number of reasons for this appearance. Head circumference is on the upper limits of normal, and achondroplastic children usually have a broad, prominent forehead with often a larger than normal lower jaw. The bridge of the nose is often flattened, and this feature adds to the optical illusion of a top-heavy head. By contrast, the base of the skull and the foramen magnum are small. This latter fact can sometimes cause compression of the spinal cord in this region, giving rise to respiratory problems. Some achondroplastic children have died suddenly and unexpectedly from this cause. Hydrocephalus, due to the abnormalities of the foramen magnum at the base of the skull, occurs in a few children with achondroplasia. This condition, too, will add to the disproportionate size of the head.

The **pelvis,** if X-rays are taken, has abnormal features. The roof of the hip-joint is flat with a protruding bony spike. This bone structure can account, in part, for the unusual waddling gait of many people with achondroplasia, although the fact of having very short legs also makes for an unusual walking pattern—especially when a person with achondroplasia tries to keep up with long-legged companions!

The normal curves of the **spine** are accentuated. The lower lumbar curve is more marked than usual. This curvature has little effect during childhood, but it can give rise to lower back pain later in life.

Eventual **height** rarely reaches more than 55 inches (140 centimeters).

Hands are broad and short, with their lack of length resulting from the shortness of the metacarpals (from wrist to knuckles). Fingers are of normal length. The achondroplastic child cannot close his/her fingers together; they remain widely spaced in spite of all his/her efforts to approximate them.

Children with achondroplasia are often **hypotonic.** Due to this condition, they are often late in sitting and starting to walk. It is inadvisable to put too much pressure on them to hurry these skills along, as the combination of weak muscles and a large head puts a great strain on the spine, with the probable effect of increasing the lordosis in the lumbar region. **Mental abilities** fall within the normal range, and intellectual abilities can be high. Most achondroplastic children are psychologically well adjusted to their small size, but problems with body image can occasionally occur.

Ears: frequent middle ear infections are common. A conductive deafness can occur later in life, due to the repeated ear infections. Sensorineural deafness can also occur.

MANAGEMENT IMPLICATIONS

The implications revolve largely around the short stature and its associated problems.

Short stature: problems with this aspect of achondroplasia will increase as the child matures. During infancy and the toddler years, lack of height is not too noticeable, but around the early school years it becomes obvious when the achondroplastic child stands next to his/her peers. Orthopedic treatments to lengthen limbs have been available in recent years. Much thought by the child and the family will need to be taken before embarking upon this long treatment, but the child may gain much confidence when several inches can be added to height. Some children have been given growth hormone at appropriate times during the growing years, but it has been recently discovered that severe problems have arisen in later years following this treatment.

Practical aids, such as suitable seating, low shelves for storage of personal possessions, smaller sports equipment, and general low-level living devices can make the life of the achondroplastic child easier. From the teenage years on, difficulties with high steps and driving problems will arise, and help must be given wherever possible.

Emotional effects, both on the affected child and the family, must not be forgotten. Parents of normal height can become greatly distressed by their child's difficulties, and where the inheritance is obvious, the parent also affected can suffer from guilt reactions. Sensitive counseling of the whole family, with time granted so the family can think through all the implications of short stature in particular, should be available. Care must also be taken to ensure that the child with achondroplasia is not treated as younger than his/her chronological age. It is all too easy to forget that in all aspects of development, other than height, the child is exactly the same as his or her peers, with similar needs—and, of course, potentially with similar behavior. (This observation applies equally to all children of short stature.)

Orthopedic abnormalities can result from abnormalities in the spine. "Slipped discs" in the lower lumbar region are not uncommon in later life, and they must be appropriately treated, probably by surgery.

Leg lengthening operations and operations to correct excessively bowed legs can be undertaken in selected cases, and such surgeries will do much to improve the quality of life. Watch must be kept for spinal cord compression weakness and tingling in lower limbs due to the abnormality in the region of the foramen magnum. Most importantly, breathing patterns must be watched carefully during childhood.

Hearing: the frequent attacks of otitis media must be treated quickly and adequately. Hearing assessment following attacks of infection should be carried out to determine if hearing has been affected by the infectious process. Myringotomy may need to be performed to counteract conductive deafness.

THE FUTURE

Persons with achondroplasia have a normal life span, and they are generally healthy individuals, as long as spinal abnormalities are not severe. Symptoms of spinal cord compression (for example, weakness, pain, or tingling in arms or legs) must be investigated urgently and treated. Job prospects are limited only by the individual's lack of inches, as intellectual ability should not be affected. With recent legal and social advances with regard to the equal treatment of disabled persons, career opportunities show more promise.

Achondroplasia is no bar to conception and pregnancy, although in most cases the delivery of the baby of a woman with achondroplasia will need to be by cesarean section due to the mother's pelvic abnormalities. Genetic counseling is advisable before embarking on a planned pregnancy. There is a 50% chance of the condition being inherited if one parent is achondroplastic and a 75% chance if both parents have the bone disorder.

HYPOCHONDROPLASIA

This is a modified form of achondroplasia in which only a certain part of the condition is present. In children with this disorder, it is the upper parts of both arms and legs that are disproportionately short—the remainder of the body and limbs being of normal size and proportions.

Short stature is also a feature of this condition, but it will not be as marked as in achondroplasia. Final height is rarely more than 5 feet 5 inches.

Inheritance patterns are the same as for achondroplasia, there being a 50% chance of the child having the condition if one parent has hypochondroplasia.

SELF-HELP GROUP

The Human Growth Foundation
997 Glen Cove Avenue
Glen Head, NY 11545
800-451-6434
http://www.hgfound.org
email: hgfl@hgfound.org

Aicardi Syndrome

INCIDENCE

The incidence of Aicardi syndrome is not known, but as the definitive triad of signs are recognized, it may be discovered that this syndrome is not as rare as was originally supposed. Only girls are affected due to the mode of inheritance, and all races seem to be involved. Certain criteria for a diagnosis of Aicardi syndrome have recently been described. Similar signs and symptoms occur in other conditions, and it is probable that persons with these other conditions are, at times, confused with individuals truly suffering from Aicardi syndrome.

This syndrome is closely associated with agenesis of the corpus collosum, in which the part of the brain linking the two cerebral hemispheres fails to develop properly. Agenesis of the corpus collosum can occur alone, giving rise to variable symptoms ranging from normality to severe learning difficulties with convulsions as an added problem. The following description applies to the abnormalities found in Aicardi syndrome.

HISTORY

In the late 1960s, Dr. Aicardi described in the French literature a recognizable set of signs and symptoms now known as Aicardi syndrome. By 1980, more than 100 patients had been identified. In 1982, the genetic basis for the syndrome was reported.

CAUSATION

At the present state of knowledge, Aicardi syndrome seems to arise due to chromosomal abnormality of the X chromosome. It is probable that this abnormality most usually occurs as a new mutation, as there has only been one report of a family with two children with the same condition. Only girls are affected, as the condition seems to be incompatible with life in the male fetus.

At present, prenatal diagnosis is not possible.

INVESTIGATIONS

EEG (electroencephalogram), CAT (computer axial tomography) scan, and MRI (magnetic resonance imaging) will aid in the diagnosis of the part of this syndrome associated with agenesis of the corpus collosum.

CHARACTERISTICS

Infantile spasms are one of the invariable characteristics of Aicardi syndrome. These are seizures of a specific type that begin in early infancy:. These spasms can occur many times during the course of the day, and they are sometimes known as "salaam attacks" due to the position taken by the baby during a seizure—rather like a formal bow. (Hypsarrhythmia is another name for these seizures.) In persons with Aicardi syndrome, this type of convulsion continues to occur in a modified form throughout life. These continual seizures are very damaging to brain function, occurring as they do with such frequency.

The EEG features of Aicardi syndrome are unusual and quite unique. There is obvious independent activity of the two halves of the brain on the tracing. It has been suggested that this distinctive finding may be due, in part, to the absence, or gross abnormality, of a specific part of the brain—the corpus callosum.

Eye abnormalities: the whole eye is often small, but the particular abnormality of the eye in Aicardi syndrome is the appearance of the retina. When viewed with an ophthalmoscope, a number of "punched out" areas are seen in this vital part of the eye. Given this condition, one might expect blindness to be inevitable, but not every person with Aicardi syndrome experiences a total loss of vision, although their sight is restricted. Nevertheless, these individuals frequently do become blind as they get older.

Brain abnormalities can be seen on CAT scans and magnetic resonance imaging. Specific areas of the brain—the corpus callosum, especially—are affected. This feature results in severe **developmental delay** and **mental retardation.** All aspects of development are affected, including large and fine movements as well as speech. Restricted vision also adds to the problems of fine movements.

Seizures and the consequences of eye and brain abnormalities are the major problems that affect all sufferers from Aicardi syndrome. Other abnormalities are also commonly seen, but they are not always present.

The **spinal column** often shows fused vertebrae or only partially developed vertebrae. As a result, **scoliosis** frequently occurs, giving rise to respiratory problems due to restricted breathing movements. This picture is made worse by ribs being often misshapen or sometimes absent altogether, placing the whole function of the chest—both heart and lungs—under stress.

Deformities of the **hands** can be present. The size of the baby's **head** can be small, and it does not show the usual continuing growth. The head circumference (a routine measurement in all babies that indicates brain development) is frequently on the lower line of the growth charts.

Expressive speech is often absent, but some persons with the syndrome can understand speech.

Sleep can be a problem, with constant waking at intervals throughout the night. This difficulty sleeping may be due to the occurrence of frequent seizures.

MANAGEMENT IMPLICATIONS

Seizures: these are especially difficult to control. Some individuals have been prescribed as many as seven different anticonvulsants to control the seizures. ACTH (adrenocorticotropic hormone) has been used to good effect, particularly when given to the infant in the early months. It is thought that early control of seizures, as far as is possible, may help to reduce further brain dysfunction.

Visual problems: the exact extent of the visual loss is difficult to diagnose accurately, due both to the anatomical effects in the retina and to the mental handicap found in children with Aicardi syndrome. Little help can be given due to the patchy loss of retinal tissue, as that tissue is vital for normal vision.

Developmental delay and **mental retardation** are profound, and the child will need full-time skilled help as he/she matures. Few children with Aicardi syndrome develop any speech. Walking is usually achieved, but it can be very late in occurring. Self-help skills, such as feeding and dressing, will be only slowly, if ever, achieved. Schools for profoundly handicapped pupils will be necessary.

The advice of a speech therapist is of value, especially if there is thought to be some difficulty in the comprehension of language.

Children with Aicardi syndrome seem to be especially prone to coughs and colds. These infections can often extend to the lower respiratory tract, giving rise to bronchitis or pneumonia. The relative immobility of the child is not helpful in preventing these complications.

THE FUTURE

The future is bleak for persons suffering from Aicardi syndrome. Full-time care will need to be given throughout life. Control of seizures will be a lifelong problem, and many children succumb to respiratory tract infections.

Because the description of Aicardi syndrome is of such recent origin, there are no substantiated reports as to how long these children can be expected to live. The oldest known survivor was 15 years old in 1989.

SELF-HELP GROUP

Aicardi Syndrome Foundation
450 Winterwood Drive
Roselle, IL 60172
800-374-8518
http://www.aicardi.com

Albinism

Albinism is a rare condition. There are a number of variants, which affect individuals differently. Many affected people have to lead an altered lifestyle due to their albinism. It is thought to occur in approximately 1 in 200,000 people overall. Albinism occurs in all races, being more common in some peoples than others. For example, the incidence in France is 1 in 100,000, while the incidence among the San Blas Indians of Panama is 7 in 1,000.

There are a number of other syndromes that have albinism as part of their characteristics.

HISTORY

Albinos, the name by which people with albinism are frequently known, have been recognized for centuries. The name was originally applied by the Portuguese to white African negroes.

The name is also applied to animals and plants lacking pigment.

CAUSATION

Albinism is a genetically inherited disease; most forms are transmitted in an autosomal recessive manner. The basic fault is one of an inborn error of metabolism: the enzyme tyrosinase is defective, and as a result, melanin—the pigment giving color to eyes, hair, and skin—is not produced, even though there are normal numbers of pigment-forming cells (melanocytes) in the basal layer of the skin.

There are several different types of albinism, which can be difficult to distinguish clinically. In one type, there may be some pigmented nevi on the body, and the hair may be yellow instead of white, suggesting that in this particular type there is some tyrosinase activity.

Albinism may be partial, so that the full effects of complete melanin lack are not seen. Very blond children with fine, delicate skin that burns easily on exposure to the sun probably have a minimal form of albinism. A type of albinism can be part of the clinical pattern of two further syndromes—Waardenburg syndrome, which is associated with deafness, and Chediak–Higashi syndrome, which has blood and immunological problems associated with the condition. Eyes alone can be affected—ocular albinism—and this type is thought most likely to be inherited in an X-linked manner.

Prenatal diagnosis is only possible by biopsy of the fetal skin, which is rarely done.

CHARACTERISTICS

Skin: albinos have very fair skin, which, without the protection of the necessary melanin, burns very readily in sunlight. Along with this fair skin goes white, silky hair. Eyebrows, eyelashes, and other body hair are also white.

Eyes: the iris is very pale, pink or blue in color. The redness of the retina can sometimes be seen through this translucent iris. As a result of this, photophobia (dislike of light) is common. Abnormalities in the visual pathways are always present in true albinism. These problems are caused by defective prenatal development of optic fibers and by poor formation of part of the retina due to lack of pigment. The abnormalities lead to much reduced vision.

Nystagmus—rapid backwards and forwards movement of the eyes—can also be present in ocular albinism. Strangely enough, nystagmus does not interfere too much with vision, although some children develop an unusual head posture in an effort to compensate for the flickering of their eyes. Nystagmus usually improves with advancing years. Lazy eye can also be present, although not invariably so.

MANAGEMENT IMPLICATIONS

Skin: very great care needs to be taken with albino children in sunlight. Even cloudy days can cause burning if the skin is exposed. Protective clothing is essential at all times, and adequate sunscreen is advisable. In hot sunny countries, the problems can be acute.

Eyes: vision must be checked on a regular basis, and corrective lenses prescribed as far as is possible. It is especially important that school-age children should receive yearly visual checks. Vision can deteriorate rapidly during periods of rapid growth in all children, and albino children are especially at risk. It is frequently not possible to obtain perfect vision, due to the eye developmental abnormality that is always present in complete albinism. Vision does not deteriorate with age. Due to the lack of protective pigment in the iris, dark glasses are often necessary to protect the eyes from light. Lazy eye, when present, should be corrected orthoptically or surgically so as to maximize all possible vision.

Early correction of lazy eye is vital if amblyopia—lack of vision in one eye—is to be avoided.

Education: about 20% of albino children will need special educational facilities due to their visual problems. These children are not completely blind, although their vision is limited enough to come within the legal definition of blindness. Emphasis in schools should be put on those activities at which the children can do well. Other children with fewer visual problems will be able to attend mainstream schools, but care of their sensitive skin must always be taken.

THE FUTURE

Albinism does not restrict life span. However, career prospects can be limited. Work outside in all weather has to be avoided due to the skin problems.

In many cases, restricted distance vision will make obtaining a driving license a problem. Near vision, however, is usually good, so careers needing fine, close work are most suitable, especially when these kind of jobs also involve inside work, where skin problems can be avoided.

Children with normally pigmented skin can be born to a couple who both have albinism. Genetic counseling should be given due to the number of variants of the condition. Careful scrutiny of family trees, identifying ancestors with very pale skin and fair hair as well as other abnormalities, will give clues as to possible inheritance patterns.

Skin cancers can arise more readily due to the lack of protective melanin. Therefore, any patch of skin that shows signs of permanent reddening, soreness, or excess itching should receive immediate attention.

SELF-HELP GROUP

NOAH
The National Organization for Albinism and Hypopigmentation
1530 Locust Street, #29
Philadelphia, PA 19102-4415
215-545-2322 or 800-473-2310
http://www.albinism.org

Albright Syndrome

ALTERNATIVE NAMES

Albright hereditary osteodystrophy (AHO); pseudohypoparathyroidism.

INCIDENCE

Albright syndrome is a rare condition. The exact number of children affected is unknown, but the condition is well documented. Basically, this syndrome arises from a fault in calcium and phosphate metabolism in the body, which in turn is due to faulty parathyroid hormone activity. Both boys and girls can be affected, but girls are more commonly seen with the syndrome.

The biochemical abnormality need not give rise to symptoms and can be found in totally asymptomatic and clinically normal people. The abnormality is only discovered when specific routine testing is undertaken in relatives of children who have Albright syndrome.

HISTORY

In 1942 Albright first recognized that the syndrome is due to a failure of the action of the parathyroid hormone on calcium and phosphates in the body. Research continued, and in 1980 the basic molecular defects of the disease were described.

CAUSATION

Albright syndrome is a genetic disorder with some uncertainties still existing as to the exact mode of inheritance. It may be that the syndrome is X-linked, which would account for the higher incidence in girls. However, other authorities consider Albright syndrome to be inherited as an autosomal dominant characteristic, but with sex modifications.

CHARACTERISTICS

Albright syndrome may not be recognized until mid-childhood, although seizures due to the altered calcium and phosphate levels can occur in infancy, when the diagnosis can be made. The following characteristics are found in the complete syndrome in mid-childhood.

Short stature: this is not usually as marked as in many other syndromes (e.g., Turner syndrome). Body proportions are normal, with legs and arms in keeping with the rest of the body. Most people with Albright syndrome reach a final height of around 5 feet, which is a quite acceptable height for most activities.

Obesity occurs commonly and makes the lack of inches appear more obvious. Albright children typically have plump, round faces with a short neck. This tendency to excessive weight gain can be noted before birth, and many babies with Albright syndrome have a high birth weight. Weight gain is rapid in the first few months. (Although the above picture of height and weight is usual in Albright syndrome, these measurements can be within the normal range.)

Skeletal system: due to the abnormalities in calcium and phosphate metabolism, unusual calcification can occur in parts of the skeleton. For example, hips and the pelvis, as well as limb bones, can have abnormal bony configurations.

Short fourth and fifth fingers are a fairly constant finding and can help in confirming the diagnosis. The shortness of these fingers is very specific and is due to the relative shortness of the terminal bones of these digits.

Eyes: cataracts can occur in Albright syndrome, although this condition is not invariably found.

Mental retardation: intelligence is sometimes normal in children with Albright syndrome, but the usual range of IQ is between 20 and 99, with a mean level of 60. The level of intelligence would seem to depend upon blood levels of calcium and phosphate. Those children with low levels of these substances are more likely to have a degree of retardation than are children with normal levels.

Thyroid under-activity is more commonly found in children with Albright syndrome than in the general population. It is important that this condition is diagnosed early if present, so that treatment with thyroid hormone can be given. It is thought probable that early treatment of this problem reduces the incidence of possible mental retardation.

MANAGEMENT IMPLICATIONS

Hypocalcemia: if low levels of blood calcium are found, treatment with vitamin D has been found to be effective. Calcium supplements may be necessary, as may other drugs to reduce the amount of calcium excreted.

Hypothyroidism must be treated with replacement thyroid hormone if levels of this hormone are found to be low. A child known to have Albright syndrome should be watched for signs of hypothyroidism, such as weight gain, slow speech, a hoarse voice, scanty hair, and dry skin. Blood levels can then confirm the clinical diagnosis.

Dietary measures to reduce obesity should be undertaken (and kept up!). The help of a dietitian should be enlisted, as it is important that nutrition is adequate for proper growth and development. Dietitians, too, have a wealth of skills that make eating the right foods fun rather than restrictive. Overweight children can suffer miseries at school. As well as being the target for teasing, they find it difficult to join in physical activities, and they are often the last person to be asked to join a team. Excess weight also puts unwanted strain on growing joints, and there may be a link between obesity and hypertension in later life. Therefore, all efforts should be made to keep weight gain to a minimum.

Learning difficulties, if present, may mean that the child will need special schooling and extra help later in childhood. Routine developmental checks and, later, school performance tests, will determine if there are any problems. Children of normal intelligence with Albright syndrome are perfectly able to cope with mainstream schooling. Care must be taken, however, that dietary regimes and any necessary medication are strictly controlled.

Eyes: cataracts will need ophthalmic assessment and treatment if present. Routine visual tests should be done to identify problems early. Good lighting and some form of magnification can be helpful to the child before any necessary operative procedures are undertaken.

Genetic counseling needs to be available for the person with Albright syndrome when the reproductive years are reached.

THE FUTURE

A normal life span is to be expected in adults with Albright syndrome. However, watch should be kept on blood pressure during adult years as severe hypertension is found in more than half of the adults with this condition. This condition can predispose a person to strokes and/or coronary artery disease. Therefore, treatment should be given to maintain blood pressure within normal limits as far as possible. Weight control will lessen the risks of hypertension. Pregnant women with this condition frequently require cesarean sections, due to the bony abnormalities in their pelvises.

SELF-HELP GROUP

There is no specific group dedicated to Albright syndrome, but relevant medical information may be obtained from:

Metabolic Information Network
P.O. Box 670847
Dallas TX 75367-0847
214-696-2188
email: mizesg@ix.netcom.com

Alport Syndrome

ALTERNATIVE NAMES

Hereditary nephritis; Fechtner syndrome.

INCIDENCE

The severity of Alport syndrome can differ widely from individual to individual. This variation may be, in part, due to the way in which the disease is inherited. Alport syndrome has been reported from many parts of the world, but, up to 1989, there were no reported cases in black children. Depending on which inherited pattern is at work, incidence is either the same in both sexes or there is a preponderance of girls suffering from the condition.

Alport syndrome is thought to be responsible for up to one-sixth of the cases of specific renal disease. Alport syndrome should always be suspected if a number of family members suffer from both renal disease and deafness.

CAUSATION

Alport syndrome is inherited in an X-linked manner. Boys with the condition are usually more severely affected than are girls, although with this form of inheritance twice as many girls are thought to be affected.

The syndrome can also be inherited as an autosomal dominant characteristic. Under these circumstances, equal numbers of boys and girls are affected. The Fechtner variant is inherited in this manner.

CHARACTERISTICS

All sufferers from Alport syndrome will have **nephritis** to some degree. Nephritis is manifested by the passage of blood and/or protein in the urine. It is more usual for these signs to appear in mid-childhood, although the pathological changes in the kidneys have been present from the early days of life. Occasionally, bouts of mild **fever** occur in association with the progressive damage to the kidneys.

At the onset of the disease, kidney function is normal. However, over the years kidney function will gradually deteriorate until, in the most severely affected, renal failure can occur during the teenage years. Under these conditions, the waste products of metabolism will not be removed adequately from the body. The child will become progressively tired and listless and have a poor appetite. Thirst will be a problem, and large quantities of dilute urine will be passed—a younger child may begin wetting the bed.

In around half of the cases of Alport syndrome, there will be **sensorineural deafness.** Deafness is found more commonly in boys; it can be slowly progressive until little residual hearing remains. Any child with recognized renal disease should be carefully checked for hearing loss. Deafness may develop as early as three to four years of age.

These two groups of symptoms are the main features of Alport syndrome, but the following added problems can occur:

- Around 15% of children will have **visual** problems—the formation of cataracts being the most common of these.
- A specific type of skin condition, known as **icthyosis,** can occur in some children with Alport syndrome. The skin, as the name implies, will be dry and scaly, like fish scales.
- A specific **blood disorder**—thrombocytopenia—in which there is a low platelet count can affect the child. This disorder can lead to numerous small patches of bruising on the child's body.

As the inevitable **renal failure** progresses, the following events can occur at varying times:

- The child will become **anemic.** Anemia is due both to the child's poor appetite and also to a reduction in the production of red blood cells.
- Raised **blood pressure** can occur as a result of the disease process in the kidneys.
- **Bony changes** similar to those seen in rickets can occur. These changes are primarily due to the kidney disease leading to a decreased absorption of calcium.
- **Growth** can be retarded by all these factors associated with the renal disease.

MANAGEMENT IMPLICATIONS

The most important aspect in the management of Alport syndrome is the maintenance of renal function. Once the diagnosis has been made, regular visits to a pediatric nephrologist (a pediatrician with a special interest in conditions of the renal tract) will be necessary. Clinical examination along with blood and urine tests and specialized X-rays and ultrasound examination will give clues as to kidney function. Depending on the results of tests, various types of drugs and nutritional regimens will be needed to counteract anemia, hypertension, and the bony changes that may occur.

Dialysis of one form or another will eventually be necessary for the person suffering from Alport syndrome. The most usual age for this treatment to become necessary is between 10 and 15 years of age. The specific reasons for starting on this form of treatment will vary from child to child. Some children will need urgent treatment following an intercurrent infection with which their kidneys cannot cope. In other instances, blood tests will show serious imbalances in the chemical composition of the blood that cannot be controlled by drugs or nutritional changes. There are three methods of dialysis that clear the waste products of metabolism from the body:

- **Hemodialysis,** in which waste products are removed from the blood. This method requires a several hour stay at a dialysis unit two or three times a week.
- **Continuous peritoneal dialysis,** in which waste products are removed from the peritoneal cavity of the abdomen. This method will need attention four times daily, but it has the advantage that the child is able to lead a more normal daily life without the need for frequent visits to a dialysis unit.
- **Continuous cycling peritoneal dialysis.** The principles applied with this method of removing waste products are similar to continual peritoneal dialysis, but here the treatment is carried out— at night—once every 24 hours. With this method, there is less disturbance of family lifestyle than the six, hourly bag changes necessary with the former method.

Dialysis of any type needs a skilled team in a specialized renal unit to oversee the initial set up of the most suitable method, and progress must be monitored continuously. Life will obviously be difficult for the whole family when dialysis is an everyday necessity.

Kidney transplantation is the ultimate aim. A transplant will, of course, relieve all need for dialysis, and once the critical period for rejection of the new kidney is over, the child will be able to lead a normal life again.

Another major problem to be considered is the progressive **deafness** from which children with Alport syndrome can suffer. Regular checking of hearing is necessary, and specialized teaching must be arranged if deafness becomes profound.

Vision also must be checked regularly, and appropriate treatment given if cataracts should be found to be developing.

Schooling may be problematic at those times when frequent hospital admissions are necessary. Health and education authorities will need to work together to provide the best facilities for the child.

Careers for children with Alport syndrome will depend very much on the severity of the disease. When renal function is minimally affected (as is sometimes the case with girls with this condition) or kidney function is restored by kidney transplantation, any career is possible. Deafness, if present, may lead to further difficulties. Good career advice from someone conversant with all the possible problems associated with this syndrome is vital for the young person.

THE FUTURE

The future will depend upon the severity of the renal disease. Boys fare worse than girls in this respect, and renal failure is frequently fatal before the age of 30 years unless kidney transplantation has been successfully undertaken. Girls often have a normal life span, in spite of kidney abnormalities being present.

SELF-HELP GROUPS

National Kidney Foundation
30 East 33rd Street, Suite 1100
New York, NY 10016
800-622-9010 or 212-889-2210
http://www.kidney.org
email: info@kidney.org

American Society of Deaf Children (ASDC)
2848 Arden Way, Suite 210
Sacramento, CA 95825-1373
800-942-2732 or 916-482-0120
email: ASDC1@aol.com

National Association of the Deaf (NAD)
814 Thayer Avenue
Silver Springs, MD 20910-4500
301-587-1788

Angelman Syndrome

ALTERNATIVE NAME

Formerly known as "happy puppet" syndrome.

INCIDENCE

The exact number of children with Angelman syndrome is not known, but more than 80 definite cases have been reported in the literature.

HISTORY

Children with Angelman syndrome were previously described as suffering from "happy puppet" syndrome, due to the rather jerky movements seen in association with outbursts of laughter. This name has now been dropped because more knowledge has been gained regarding the genetic basis for this condition.

CAUSATION

Angelman syndrome is a chromosomal disorder, the faulty chromosome being chromosome 15. There has been found to be a deletion in the same region of this chromosome as is seen in Prader–Willi syndrome. In spite of this similarity, the two syndromes are clinically very different. It is thought that the problem in the case of Angelman syndrome is derived from the maternal side, while the defect in Prader–Willi syndrome is considered to arise from the father. In most cases, this syndrome occurs out of the blue, although five families have been reported to have two children with the same condition.

Angelman syndrome is not evident at birth, but it becomes obvious as the child matures. Prenatal tests are available under certain specific circumstances, but such examinations are not applicable to every family. If possible, parents should receive genetic counseling before embarking upon another pregnancy.

CHARACTERISTICS

Microcephaly: at birth, the baby's head circumference is within normal limits. As the child grows, this important measurement is seen to fall behind the other parameters of growth, and the head never reaches normal size.

During infancy, **feeding** can be a problem, largely due to poor brain development causing difficulties in sucking.

Normal **sleep patterns** are often difficult to establish. Babies with Angelman syndrome are frequently hyperactive, and they seem to need little sleep—and only at inappropriate times!

Developmental delay leading to severe **mental retardation** occurs over the early years. Babies up to approximately one year of age can appear to be progressing normally, but from then on, they show signs of delayed development. The following problems are particularly common:

- **Speech** is affected to a disproportionate degree. Expressive speech is never properly attained, although receptive language develops, enabling children with Angelman syndrome to understand simple commands.
- **Walking** is late, and a typical jerky gait in noticeable in the early years, although the gait does tend to improve in later childhood. The unusual gait occasionally produces deformities in joints, which may need correction at a later date.
- **Arm movements** are also jerky and repetitive.
- **Hand flapping,** often associated with outbursts of inappropriate laughter, is another obvious characteristic. The laughter is not thought to be connected with epilepsy—as can be the case in certain conditions—but rather due to involuntary motor activity.
- **Seizures** are common during infancy and childhood, and a characteristic pattern is seen on EEG tracing. These seizures may decrease spontaneously in later life.
- **Facial features:** children with Angelman syndrome tend to have large mouths with widely spaced teeth. Tongues tend to protrude, and this feature is especially noticeable during the outbursts of laughter.

Children with Angelman syndrome are usually happy and affectionate young people. One of the greatest problems associated with this syndrome is the child's inability to speak. In spite of this handicap, children appear to enjoy life and seem especially to enjoy music and activities involving water.

MANAGEMENT IMPLICATIONS

Feeding and **sleep** problems early in life, along with a degree of **hyperactivity,** will need attention. Small, frequent meals and a regular routine in an attempt to rationalize the sleeping pattern is the best method of approach. These practices can take much patience and support. Short-term sedation may be necessary to break the difficult sleeping pattern and to allow the parents to get some sleep themselves.

Speech therapy help is indicated as the speech problems become obvious. Nonverbal techniques of communication such as sign language may help to relieve some of the frustration felt by the child who lacks usual communication skills. It is rare that any understandable speech is ever attained.

Seizures will need to be controlled with anticonvulsants. The dosage and type of anticonvulsant will need to be checked on a regular basis as seizures tend to reduce naturally later in childhood.

Mental retardation will require educational facilities designed for severely handicapped pupils, where there is an emphasis on training in self-help skills. This training will need to be continued in a suitable environment after the child has passed statutory school age.

THE FUTURE

Regrettably, children with Angelman syndrome will never be able to lead an independent life. Full-time care will be necessary, preferably in a warm, loving environment where some degree of suitable communication can take place.

Life expectancy is thought to be normal. There have been no reports of children being born to persons with Angelman syndrome.

SELF-HELP GROUP

Angelman Syndrome Foundation (ASF)
414 Plaza Drive, Suite 209
Westmont, IL 60559
800-432-6435 or 630-734-9267
http://ww-chem.ucsd.edu/asf/index.html
email: asf@adminsys.com

Ankylosing Spondylitis

INCIDENCE

The incidence of ankylosing spondylitis in children is comparatively rare. It is less common than rheumatoid arthritis, with which it can easily be confused in the early stages. Caucasian populations have a higher incidence than either Japanese or black African peoples, in whom the condition is rare.

Symptoms usually first occur in the later childhood years, but children as young as five years have been known to suffer from ankylosing spondylitis.

The condition is found more commonly in boys than in girls.

CAUSATION

Ankylosing spondylitis has an autosomal inheritance in families who have a specific antigen in their white blood cells known as HLA-B27, and chromosome 6 is the site on which the faulty gene is found. However, only a relatively small percentage (around 20 to 25%) of children with this antigen in their blood will develop the condition. Interaction with specific infections may have a bearing on the development of the disease.

There is no prenatal diagnosis possible at the present time.

CHARACTERISTICS

The spine is the main part of the skeleton affected in ankylosing spondylitis. **Lower back pain** with stiffness of movement, especially when getting out of bed in the morning, will be the most usual early sign.

In some children, however, the initial feature will be **inflammatory, arthritic-type pain** in one or more of the lower limb joints—the hip or the knee. This feature can make it difficult for doctors to differentiate this condition from other forms of arthritis.

As the disease progresses, the normal forward bend of the spine in the lower back (lumbar lordosis) is lost. The upper part of the spine can also become involved, and the child will develop a **stooping posture**. (This latter feature occurs in the most severe form of the disease. Many children—and adults—only have the lower part of their back involved.)

For a small number of children with ankylosing spondylitis, inflammation in a specific part of the **eye** can occur. This condition can precede, or accompany, the features seen in the skeletal system.

It is important that a correct diagnosis is made as soon as possible so that treatment to alleviate the effects of this condition can begin.

INVESTIGATIONS

X-ray of the spine will show specific changes, including the complete fusion together of the affected vertebrae in the advanced stages.

Blood tests will be negative for the rheumatoid factor, but in practically all cases the antigen HLA-B27 will be present.

MANAGEMENT IMPLICATIONS

Anti-inflammatory drugs to relieve the pain caused by the initial inflammatory stage of the disease will be necessary. The need for such drugs will diminish as the affected vertebrae become fused together.

Physical therapy is a vital, ongoing part of treatment both to maintain joint mobility and to maintain, as far as possible, a normal posture. A stooping, rounded back will automatically put a strain on other joints and muscles, giving rise to further pain and immobility.

Hydrotherapy, with graded exercises undertaken in warm water, can be particularly helpful. The water helps to support the body, thus making movement freer and less painful.

Schooling can be in mainstream schools as long as the teaching staff are aware of the child's difficulties in movement. Affected children should be allowed to choose for themselves whether or not they are able to participate in games or other physical exercise. Allowance must also be made for absences from school for physical therapy sessions.

Any **inflammation of the eyes** should receive immediate medical attention.

THE FUTURE

A normal life span can be expected, and with adequate and suitable treatment, a normal lifestyle can be followed. However, children with ankylosing spondylitis should be guided toward careers with less physical, more sedentary, components.

SELF-HELP GROUP

Spondylitis Association of America (SAA)
14827 Ventura Blvd., Suite 119
P.O. Box 5872
Sherman Oaks, CA 91403
818-981-1616 or 800-777-8189
http://www.spondylitis.org
email: spondy@aol.com

Apert Syndrome

ALTERNATIVE NAMES

Acrocephalosyndactyly type 1; Vogt cephalosyndactyly.

INCIDENCE

Apert syndrome is one of the most serious conditions in a group of syndromes known as acrocephalosyndactyly, which are characterized by premature fusion of the bones of the skull, together with malformations of the hands and feet. The condition is rare, only occurring in between 1 in 100,000 and 1 in 160,000 births. Both boys and girls can be affected, and the condition can be diagnosed at birth.

CAUSATION

Apert syndrome can be inherited as autosomal dominant. But few cases of direct inheritance from either parent are known. Most of the cases seem to arise as new mutations. There have been suggestions that older fathers may be more at risk of having a child with Apert syndrome, but this hypothesis has not been conclusively proved.

CHARACTERISTICS

The bones of the skull in new-born babies are normally separated from each other. This separation aids the process of birth as the skull is able to mold to the birth canal. Soon after birth, the edges of these flat bones become joined together by fibrous tissue in specific places. These positions of fusion are known as the "sutures" of the skull. It is at these positions that future skull growth occurs to accommodate the underlying growing brain. In Apert syndrome (and also in other syndromes of a similar nature), these sutures fuse together prematurely. This early fusion gives rise to the typical characteristics of the head and the face seen in children with this syndrome.

Head: the most striking features of babies born with Apert syndrome is their high, prominent forehead, often with a marked swelling in the mid-line. The backs of the heads of these babies tend to be more flattened than is usual.

Facial features: The lower jaw is often large, while the nose is small and flattened. The nasal abnormalities can give rise to both breathing and feeding difficulties in the neonatal period. Eyes are large and prominent, and they are usually widely set apart.

Ears tend to be low-set, and a congenital hearing loss is frequently present.

The **hands** of babies with Apert syndrome can also be malformed. The severity of this deformity can vary a good deal. Sometimes, only webbing of the skin between the fingers is present, but the worst cases show some bones of the hands (usually in the second, third, and fourth fingers) completely fused together. If severe bone fusion occurs, the hands have a claw-like appearance.

Feet are usually normal, but in rare cases they can have a similar appearance to the hands.

Mild **mental retardation** occurs in around 50% of children with Apert syndrome—the remaining 50% have normal IQs. Any slowing of abilities will gradually become apparent over the months and years and will be identified during routine developmental checks.

Hydrocephalus, caused by faulty drainage of cerebrospinal fluid in the ventricles of the brain, is a not infrequent complication of Apert syndrome.

A further complication seen in a large number of young people with this syndrome is severe **acne** during the adolescent years.

MANAGEMENT IMPLICATIONS

Initially, **feeding** and **breathing** difficulties commonly occur, as nasal abnormalities make it difficult, if not impossible, for the baby to breathe while he/she is feeding. Therefore, in the early days, nasogastric feeding will probably be necessary. Within three to four months of birth, these problems resolve themselves as the nasal passages enlarge with general growth.

If **hydrocephalus** occurs, a shunt will need to be inserted to drain the excess fluid away from the brain. This complication, so often seen in babies with Apert syndrome, can be difficult to diagnose in the early stages because the more usual signs of hydrocephalus tend to be obscured by the unusual shape of the skull. Careful checks on developmental patterns and neurological signs, such as increased tone in the lower limbs (for example), will be necessary to exclude this problem.

Surgery to correct the premature fusion of the bones of the skull must be undertaken, and the child may need a series of operations over the years. It is thought that these corrective procedures may help to prevent mental retardation. Surgery may also be necessary on hands, and sometimes feet, to achieve maximum function and for cosmetic reasons.

Regular **developmental checks** are of vital importance to diagnose early any slowing, or regression, of physical function and other skills.

Frequent stays in the hospital for various necessary operative procedures will be required, and children with Apert syndrome will need extra loving stimulation between these visits so that vital learning processes are not hindered.

Understanding and support for parents and child will need to be available, due not least to the unusual facial and limb features. Other children and adults can be particularly unkind to children who look "different."

THE FUTURE

Life expectancy for people with Apert syndrome can be normal, but it is dependent upon the degree of involvement of the central nervous system.

Career prospects can be affected by hand deformities and by limited mental abilities. Unusual facial features also make for some restrictions in work possibilities.

SELF-HELP GROUPS

Apert Support and Information Network
P.O. Box 1184
Fair Oaks, CA 95628
916-961-1092
email: apert@ix.netcom.com

Children's Craniofacial Association
P.O. Box 280297
Dallas, TX 75228
800-535-3643 or 972-994-9902
email: CHAR SMITH@prodigy.net

Arthrogryposis

INCIDENCE

There are a number of similar conditions that fall under the main heading of arthrogryposes. The full name of the most common of these conditions is arthrogryposis multiplex congenita (AMC). The next most common subgroup is probably "distal arthrogryposis," in which only the hands and feet are affected. There are a number of other variants described, all of which have similar characteristics but show some specific features. For example, in some children, weakness of the muscles is the predominant condition, while other children have greater problems with neurological involvement of certain spinal cord segments.

Around 1 baby in every 10,000 is born afflicted with the most common subgroup, AMC. Both boys and girls are equally affected.

CAUSATION

Arthrogryposes are genetically inherited conditions. Among the wide variety of known types, the inheritance pattern cannot be generalized. Distal arthrogryposis is inherited as an autosomal dominant condition, while AMC is thought to arise spontaneously as a new mutation. Therefore, it is important that the exact diagnosis is known when genetic counseling is given. In this way, more accurate predictions about whether further children will be born with the abnormality can be given.

Babies with arthrogryposis can be diagnosed at birth. Hints that fetal movements may be diminished can be confirmed by ultrasound over a specific period of time (for example, one hour). Delivery can sometimes be difficult due to the relative immobility of the baby. This traumatic delivery can, at times, lead to some degree of mental handicap.

CHARACTERISTICS

Children with any of the arthrogryposes have **joint deformities.** It is usual that many joints are affected. In distal arthrogryposis, only the joints of the lower legs and forearms are affected. All of the joint deformities occur because the soft tissues around the joints are contracted or stiffened. Due to this condition, the joints themselves are rendered almost immobile and certainly without normal, useful function.

The following conditions will affect a baby born with the severe form of the most common of the arthrogryposes, AMC.

Joint deformities: soon after birth, the baby with this form of arthrogryposis will lie in a very typical position caused by the deformities to be found in his/her joints. Shoulders will be pushed forward, with arms are rotated inward with flexed wrists and fingers turned in toward the palms of the hands. Similarly, feet are flexed into a position that resembles a "club foot" deformity.

Muscles in many cases are small and weak, often being replaced by fibrous or fatty tissue. Without adequate muscle power, joints become even more immobile. A very noticeable feature in some babies with AMC is the lack of normal elbow and/or knee creases, which is an obvious feature of most newborn babies. The unusual appearance is directly due to the lack of muscle development.

Short stature can be a feature in later life, as normal growth of bone is, in part, dependent on adequate movement, which is impossible without normal muscle. The shortness is not extreme, but it is nevertheless obvious.

Nevi: "strawberry" marks are very commonly seen in babies with AMC, particularly around the mid-line of the face and body.

In addition to the nevi, which are minor abnormalities, there can be more serious problems around the mid-line of the body and head: **defects in the abdominal wall; inguinal hernia;** and **asymmetry of the face.** Fortunately, these problems only occur in relatively few babies with AMC. Specialized care and treatment will be necessary for babies with these more severe defects.

MANAGEMENT IMPLICATIONS

It is important that the diagnosis of arthrogryposis is made early in the baby's life so that treatment to mobilize limbs, as far as possible, is started early.

Physical therapy is the mainstay of treatment, and it concentrates mainly on mobilizing any muscle tissue that is present. Passive stretching of affected limbs, with joints put gently through the full range of movement, on a regular basis, is of great value.

Splinting of affected joints in optimum position is also necessary. This treatment has to be done very carefully in order to avoid damage to the weakened muscular tissue. The advice of an orthopedic surgeon, working in close liaison with the physical therapist, is vital to ensure maximum function in the future. Maximum mobility should be the aim, so that bone growth is diminished as little as possible.

Most children with arthrogryposis manage quite adequately in **mainstream schools.** Stairs can be a problem, and children may need to uses ramps, for example, if buildings are not all on one level. Participation in physical education classes will not be possible for any but the most minimally affected children. Other suitable activities should be arranged during these classes for the child with arthrogryposis if full integration into mainstream schooling is to be achieved. An occupational therapist can give advice on occupations appropriate for those times that can also help with limb mobility.

THE FUTURE

Children with arthrogryposis can lead full, satisfying lives within the bounds of their physical limitations. Mental ability is not affected in any way by the condition, so any number of careers are open. Obviously, those activities needing physical strength or mobility are not possible, but numerous other sedentary and intellectual pursuits are options. Expected life span is not decreased by arthrogryposis.

For women with arthrogryposis, normal vaginal delivery will probably not be possible, and babies must be delivered by cesarean section.

SELF-HELP GROUP

Avenues-Arthrogryposis Multiplex Congenita
P.O. Box 5192
Sonora, CA 95370
209-928-3688
email: avenues@sonnet.com

Asperger Syndrome

INCIDENCE

The incidence of Asperger syndrome is not yet known, as no large-scale detailed studies have been carried out; however, research is continuing in this direction. The latest work seems to suggest that boys are affected around seven times more frequently than girls. The classification is somewhat confused, but at the present time, Asperger syndrome refers to children with less severe autistic features. These children can use nonemotional speech, but they show obsessional interests and tend to be clumsy. The incidence of autism is thought to be around 1 in every 2,500 live births, so Asperger syndrome is but a part of this overall incidence.

HISTORY

In 1944, Austrian psychiatrist Hans Asperger first described the characteristics of children who showed lack of social adjustment and much self-absorption. Around the same time, Dr. Kanner reported similar features but placed more emphasis on the specific speech and language problems. Dr. Lorna Wing in the UK has done much work on autism.

CAUSATION

There is no known definitive cause of either autism or Asperger syndrome. Other syndromes, such as fragile X syndrome, can show autistic features to a greater or lesser degree. Dr. Asperger theorized that this syndrome must be genetically transmitted. He noted a high incidence of similar characteristics in the fathers of those children with the syndrome. Some children—about half in one series—had some history of birth problems, leading to the conclusion that in some cases, organic brain deficiencies may be a causative factor.

CHARACTERISTICS

Six features have been noted to be present in persons suffering from Asperger syndrome.

- Grave difficulties with **interactive play** with peers. Children with Asperger syndrome do not wish to socialize and are unable to form relationships with other children. They are seen as cold, immature, or eccentric, and as a result, they are usually left to play on their own.
- Children with Asperger syndrome become **totally absorbed** in one specific hobby or aspect of life, to the exclusion of every other facet of daily living. This interest may be anything from chess to stamp collecting or astronomy, the subject often having a highly intellectual content.
- Children with this syndrome need to adhere strictly to **routine** in all aspects of daily living. They become extremely upset if their routine is upset. For example, if the child's usual bedtime is relaxed, this one minor alteration in the timetable can be very distressing for all the family.
- **Speech and language** are often repetitive, with a flat, monotonous, and often expressively perfect delivery. Comprehension of language appears to fall behind the normal expressive component. For example, jokes are often taken at their face value—with sometimes embarrassing consequences.
- The vast majority of children with Asperger syndrome show varying degrees of **clumsiness.** Actions are stiff, and often odd postures are struck.
- **Facial expression and gestures** used in association with speech are frequently inappropriate or clumsy. For example, yawning or smiling at the wrong time during a conversation is typical of the child with this syndrome.

MANAGEMENT IMPLICATIONS

It has been noted that the person with Asperger syndrome usually improves over time. After the turmoil of adolescence is over, behavior becomes more normal and acceptable. This improvement can be maximized by extra care and teaching in those specific areas that are particularly important to children with Asperger syndrome.

Social and communication skills: it is in this area of development that most difficulties are experienced. Specific efforts need to be made to teach these skills, many of which are picked up automatically by the normal child. Normal social interaction is a closed book to most children with Asperger syndrome. The normal give-and-take of socializing can be totally bewildering, and as a result, appropriate responses for different social situations will have to be learned. This skill is quite possible to achieve, given that children with Asperger syndrome characteristically like rote learning and repetitive behavior. It is important that the child is not allowed to withdraw into him- or herself to avoid social activities. This behavior is counterproductive, even if it is a very understandable way of avoiding difficult situations.

Language may be delayed, and speech therapists can pinpoint the specific areas of difficulty. For example, words that are used to describe actions (verbs) can be more of a mystery than words used to denote objects (nouns). It is important that the teaching of language takes place alongside the teaching of social skills in familiar situations. Coordinating these two aspects of the child's education will help comprehension and assist in preventing repetitive and obsessive behavior.

Behavioral therapy: dealing with the obsessive and ritualistic behavior of children with Asperger syndrome is one of the more difficult problems. The best approach is probably a graded change of behavior patterns, starting off with small steps and continuing slowly until the rituals no longer intrude into normal life.

It must always be remembered that children with this condition have difficulties forming relationships. "Coldness" and a lack of concern for other people's thoughts and feelings will probably always be a feature of the child's personality, and this facet must be taken into account when activities, and careers, are being planned.

Schooling: dealing with the disabling problems caused by Asperger syndrome is complex and demands much sensitivity. There is no one particular type of school suitable for all persons with Asperger syndrome. Some children will be able to manage in mainstream schools, while others may fare better in any one of a number of specialized facilities. Each child needs to be placed according to her or his own specific abilities.

THE FUTURE

Depending on the severity of the manifestation of Asperger syndrome, some form of employment is often possible in adult life. Work involving a regular routine is the best choice, and it is important that employers and fellow workers have a sympathetic understanding of the individual's eccentricities. Other, more severely affected, men and women, particularly those with speech and language difficulties, are unable to hold down any kind of job, so sheltered accommodation and care will be needed for life. However, even in severely affected people, a reduction in disability does seem to occur with time.

SELF-HELP GROUP

National Alliance for Autism Research
414 Wall Street, Research Park
Princeton, NJ 08540
609-430-9160 or 888-777-NAAR
http://www.naar.org
email: naar@naar.org

Ataxia Telangiectasia

ALTERNATIVE NAMES

Louis–Barr syndrome; Boder–Sedgwick syndrome.

INCIDENCE

Ataxia telangiectasia is a rare condition, affecting only 1 in every 30,000 to 50,000 babies. In some particular countries, such as Turkey, a comparatively high number of cases occurs. That higher rate of incidence is possibly due to the fact that intermarriage between close relatives is more common in those areas. Both boys and girls can be equally affected.

CAUSATION

Ataxia telangiectasia is thought to be transmitted as an autosomal recessive characteristic. This form of transmission would account for the high incidence in countries where it is more likely that parents are related. There may be other cases where the condition is due to a new mutation. Gene mapping has recently demonstrated that the ataxia telangiectasia gene is located on chromosome 11.

Prenatal testing is difficult at present, and identifying modes of inheritance strongly depends on looking at other members of the family in detail. Serum alpha-fetoprotein levels are frequently, but not invariably, raised in people with ataxia telangiectasia. Measuring these levels can help with diagnosis.

Ataxia telangiectasia is not apparent at birth and only becomes obvious between the ages of one and two, when the child starts to walk.

CHARACTERISTICS

Walking: As soon as a definite walking pattern is established, it is noticeable that the toddler is more unsteady on his/her feet than would be expected for the developmental stage reached. This unsteadiness is quite apparent after the child passes the age when tumbles are the norm for the new walker. This ataxia persists throughout life and may worsen as the child matures. Later in life, involuntary movements of limbs become apparent, much as is seen in certain types of cerebral palsy. (In ataxia

45

telangiectasia, the basic pathology is a very much reduced number of specialized [Purkinje] cells in the cerebellum, that part of the brain associated with the control of balance. As with many disorders, there may be an enzyme defect involved.)

Speech can become slurred and disjointed, due to the difficulty of control of muscular movement. After the initial period of deterioration in the preschool years, this particular problem should stabilize, and the child with ataxia telangiectasia can always be understood.

Later in life, prominent blood vessels—**telangiectases**—appear on the white part of the eyes. Little dilated vessels are seen to be coursing over the eye, rather as if the child had conjunctivitis without the surrounding inflammation seen in that infectious condition. Unlike conjunctivitis, ataxia telangiectasia does not make the eyes sore or itchy. These characteristic changes in the eye can also sometimes be seen on the ears.

Infections of all kinds are frequent, and even minor ones can be serious. This problem is due to an associated defect in the immune system of the child with ataxia telangiectasia. Respiratory infections, which can be difficult to treat adequately, are the most common type.

Malignancies, which can affect any site in the body, are more common for persons with ataxia telangiectasia than for other people. It is thought that around one-third of all ataxia telangiectasia sufferers will develop cancer at some time in their lives.

Sensitivity to radiation is a further feature of ataxia telangiectasia. This condition becomes of vital importance when radiation is needed to treat any cancerous growths that occur. Even the carefully controlled doses of radiation given to treat malignant growths almost always cause scars of fibrous tissue. (However, the low dosage of radiation used in normal X-ray examinations—for example, to diagnose the exact nature of a respiratory infection—is not harmful.)

Growth will slow in some, but not all, children with ataxia telangiectasia.

Sexual maturity is often late in being attained. This is due, in girls, to lack of ovarian growth and function.

MANAGEMENT IMPLICATIONS

Although no specific treatment can halt the course of the disease, much can be done to make life easier for persons with ataxia telangiectasia and their families.

The ataxia can occasionally be helped by the giving of **antispasmodic drugs.** The ongoing nature of the situation must eventually be appreciated, however, and a suitable lifestyle organized.

Some children will be confined to a wheelchair by their early teen years, and **schooling** has to be geared to this fact. A school for physically handicapped pupils may be needed if buildings in local mainstream schools are not suitable—lacking, for example, ramps or accessible toilet facilities.

Typewriters or **word processors** are useful if the ataxia affects hands and arms, making writing illegible. Special guards can be fitted, making it easier for the child to hit the correct keys.

Speech therapy can help young children with the proper development of verbal skills. Such therapy can do much to overcome communication problems.

Infections must be reduced to a minimum. For example, relatives and friends should be asked to stay away from the child if they think they are incubating a respiratory tract infection. It is a practical impossibility to avoid all infections in children, however, and illnesses that do occur must be treated quickly and adequately by the appropriate antibiotic.

The early stages of **cancer** must be watched for, and any suspicious symptoms should be investigated fully and quickly. In particular, any low-grade fever that continues for any length of time must be viewed seriously, as it may be due to a hidden source of infection or an early manifestation of cancerous growth. If cancer does occur, special care with radiation therapy must be taken because persons with ataxia telangiectasia are highly sensitive to this form of treatment.

THE FUTURE

Life expectancy for the child with ataxia telangiectasia is not great, and many will die in their twenties or thirties. Overwhelming infection or the results of malignant disease account for most of these tragically early deaths.

SELF-HELP GROUP

National Ataxia Foundation
2600 Fernbrook Lane, Suite 119
Minneapolis, MN 55447
612-553-0020
http://ataxia.org
email: naf@mr.net

Batten Disease

ALTERNATIVE NAME

Batten–Vogt syndrome.

INCIDENCE

Batten disease is one of a wide group of diseases that have a metabolic basis for the signs and symptoms seen. More than 1,000 of these metabolic conditions have been described. They all have in common some enzyme malfunction that results in imbalances of chemicals in the body. Signs and symptoms will be wide-ranging, depending on which system of the body is most involved. The substances involved in Batten disease (and related conditions) are the neuronal ceroid-lipofuscinoses (NCL). Batten disease has at least four main types, the age of onset of the symptoms being the main point of differentiation. It is a comparatively rare condition, although an incidence of 1 in 13,000 of the infantile type has been reported from Finland. Both boys and girls can be equally affected.

HISTORY

Many of the metabolic disorders have been known and described for years. It is only fairly recently, however, that the biochemical basis for many of these conditions has been understood. With increasing knowledge, more groups of signs and symptoms (syndromes!) are being found to be due to an enzyme malfunction.

CAUSATION

Batten disease is inherited as an autosomal recessive characteristic. The gene is located on chromosome 16, and prenatal diagnosis has been possible by amniocentesis. Genetic counseling before future pregnancies is advisable.

CHARACTERISTICS

The four different types of Batten disease are all characterized by progressive mental and physical deterioration, loss of vision, and seizures.

The extent of each of these aspects varies among the different types of the disease.

Infantile type (also known as the Santavouri or Finnish type)

This type becomes obvious at around one year of age. **Seizures** occur at this time, and a lag in **mental development** is noticed. Normal developmental abilities slow, and milestones tested by routine developmental checks fall behind the norm. The **ability to walk,** instead of gradually increasing in strength and stability, becomes more and more unsteady.

Head circumference (that excellent indicator of brain growth in the early years) fails to increase along the normal growth lines plotted on growth charts, and microcephaly becomes obvious within a year or two.

Regrettably, the course of the disease is rapidly downhill, and death usually occurs between the ages of five and ten years, most often due to some intercurrent infection.

Late infantile type (also known as Jansky–Bielchowsky type)

Development proceeds normally until two to four years of age. At around this time, **seizures** occur, which become more and more difficult to control.

The child's **walking** becomes increasingly clumsy and ataxic, and fine motor movements are also affected. Many of the skills already learned in both these areas of development become increasingly difficult for the child to perform.

Along with these problems goes an increasing **visual loss,** which is due to a degeneration of the retina that results directly from the enzyme defect. Nothing can be done to halt this process, and the child will eventually lose most of his/her vision.

Mental deterioration occurs, and skills previously learned are lost.

As with the infantile form, death occurs in childhood, usually by ten years of age, and, again, an intercurrent infection is the most common cause.

Juvenile NCL (also known as Speilmeyer–Vogt disease)

This type does not make its presence known until the child is between six and ten years old. The first signs of this form of Batten disease is a diminution in vision, which is due to changes in the pigment of the retina. As a result of these changes, the ability to transmit images to the brain is lost.

Within a few months of this deterioration, there is a slowing of **mental abilities,** and **seizures** occur.

The child will have **muscular coordination problems;** walking becomes ataxic; and fine hand movements become clumsy and difficult to perform. Paralysis may ultimately result.

Death occurs between the ages of 15 and 25 years.

Adult type (also known as Kufs disease)

Signs of the adult type can begin as early as puberty—when the child is around 13 to 15 years old—or the disease may not become obvious until the individual reaches her/his late twenties.

The most marked initial effects in this type are **personality changes.** The young person's behavior may become unpredictable, with outbursts of laughing or crying and other bizarre episodes. Manic phases can be especially difficult to handle, and professional guidance is valuable for parents during this time. It can, of course, be difficult to differentiate between this behavior and the often incomprehensible behavior of normal adolescence! However, in adult Batten disease, the personality changes are progressive and can end in severe dementia.

Later, in this type, problems of **balance** resulting in an ataxic gait are seen.

In marked contradistinction to the earlier forms of Batten disease, visual disturbances are not usually seen. Seizures are also not a feature of the adult type.

People with this condition can survive into middle age.

MANAGEMENT IMPLICATIONS

Control of **seizures** is one of the mainstays of medical treatment. However, seizures can be difficult to control, and often many different anticonvulsant drugs (or combinations) will need to be tried. Anti-Parkinsonian drugs can sometimes help the ataxic symptoms.

Support for the family of the child with Batten disease is of great importance. Once the diagnosis has been firmly made, parents should be counseled as to the course and final outcome of their child's condition. If at all possible, a sympathetic, knowledgeable ear should be available whenever necessary to answer queries. Such support is especially important in cases in which more than one member of the family is affected by Batten disease.

As the disease progresses, **schooling** for the older child with Batten disease will probably need to be in a special center. Continual assessment of mental abilities, as well as frequent checks on the state of the child's vision, will need to be done to provide the most suitable environment.

Recently, bone marrow transplantation in selected children has been undertaken in an attempt to halt the disease.

THE FUTURE

The future is bleak for children with the forms of Batten disease that have an early onset, as death usually occurs by the age of ten years. The forms arising later in life also have an unhappy outlook, with declining mental abilities, as well as visual problems, affecting individuals with the juvenile type. As with all handicaps, children are happiest and best cared for in a warm, loving family environment.

SELF-HELP GROUP

Batten Disease Support and Research Association (BDSRA)
2600 Parsons Avenue
Columbus, Ohio 43207-2972
800-448-4570
http://www.bdsra.org

Beckwith–Wiedemann Syndrome

ALTERNATIVE NAMES

Beckwith syndrome; EMG syndrome.

INCIDENCE

The actual incidence of Beckwith–Wiedemann syndrome is not entirely clear, but one authority suggests that 7 in 100,000 births is a probable figure. It is thought that there are a number of children with the syndrome who have not been diagnosed. Some babies born with an abnormality around the umbilicus probably also have Beckwith–Wiedemann syndrome, or at least a variant of the condition.

A much higher incidence in the West Indies has been reported—1 baby in every 13,700 is the figure quoted.

Both boys and girls are affected.

HISTORY

In 1963–64, Dr. Beckwith in the United States, and Dr. Wiedemann in France reported independently on babies with the specific characteristics associated with this syndrome. Since that time, much has been reported and written on this condition.

CAUSATION

Beckwith–Wiedemann syndrome is a genetic disorder. The exact mode of inheritance is, at present, not clear, but it is probable that the syndrome is inherited as an autosomal dominant. The syndrome is also thought to arise sporadically as a new mutation.

Ultrasonic examination can find evidence of the specific characteristics of Beckwith–Wiedemann syndrome at the 20th week of pregnancy. The abnormalities found include a defective umbilicus and enlarged kidneys.

CHARACTERISTICS

Umbilical abnormalities are seen at birth in babies with Beckwith–Wiedemann syndrome. The abnormalities can range from a small umbilical hernia to a complete failure of the muscles of the anterior abdominal wall to close together. The latter defect is severe and will urgently need surgical repair to protect the abdominal organs, which will only be covered by thin membranous tissue. (This defect is known as omphalocele.)

The **tongues** of babies with this syndrome are unusually large and protrude from the mouth. This condition can give rise to breathing problems as the enlarged tongue can fall back into the throat and impede breathing.

As the child matures, further problems can occur with **tooth eruption,** and some children with this syndrome are unable to close their top and bottom front teeth together—an "open bite." (It has been suggested that hydramnios frequently accompanies pregnancies when women are carrying fetuses with Beckwith–Wiedemann syndrome because the enlarged tongue can make it impossible for the fetus to swallow amniotic fluid.)

Birth weight is usually above average for babies with Beckwith–Wiedemann syndrome. During the first few months of life, the baby puts on weight rapidly. Growth, in terms of both height and weight, is usually along the 90th percentile on the standard growth charts. X-ray examinations show advanced bone development throughout childhood. Along with the unusual gain in weight and height goes an increased rate of growth of certain organs of the body—most usually the kidneys. The adrenals—those endocrine organs sitting on top of each kidney—are also frequently enlarged. Occasionally, there is an excessive overgrowth of a particular part of the body, such as one limb, or an entire side of the body. This excessive growth rate slows after the first few years.

Hypoglycemia (low blood sugar) in the very early days of life affects a significant number of babies with the syndrome. Symptoms of hypoglycemia include seizures, breathing and feeding problems, lethargy, and cyanosis. All these symptoms could be due to a number of conditions, but if the possible relationship between hypoglycemia and Beckwith–Wiedemann syndrome is recognized, the diagnosis can be made early. It is important that this hypoglycemia should be treated early, for it is a well-known factor in the causation of later mental handicap. The hypoglycemia is thought to be due to the overgrowth of insulin-producing cells in the pancreas.

Facial characteristics: children with Beckwith–Wiedemann syndrome tend to have small noses and rather prominent brows. At birth, and for the first year of life, flamelike nevi are often seen over the eyelids and forehead.

Ears, in many cases, have been reported to have a slight indentation on either one lobe, or on both. This indentation is one further clue to diagnosis.

Tumors of the kidney (Wilm's tumors), or of the adrenal cortex, are more likely to occur in children with this syndrome. Such tumors are probably an anomaly of the increased growth pattern seen in so many children with Beckwith–Wiedemann syndrome.

MANAGEMENT IMPLICATIONS

Umbilical abnormalities must be treated surgically with a degree of urgency if they are severe. Infection and injury are ever-present threats if the defect in the abdominal wall is large. A small umbilical hernia can, of course, be left until the baby is more mature and better able to withstand operative procedures.

Neonatal hypoglycemia must be diagnosed and treated in order to prevent mental retardation.

The enlarged **tongue** usually becomes less of a problem as the surrounding structures of the child's face grows. Orthodontic treatment for unusual "bite" patterns may be needed later in childhood. A large, soft nipple is an advantage when feeding the baby who has Beckwith–Wiedemann syndrome. In very rare cases, the tongue enlargement persists and causes breathing problems during sleep, when the tongue can fall back and block respiratory passages. Under these circumstances, an operation to reduce the size of the tongue may be necessary. Respiration may be aided by putting the baby to sleep on his/her side.

Speech therapy may occasionally be necessary to overcome the relative clumsiness of the tongue.

Watch must be kept for **tumors,** in particular Wilm's tumors, throughout childhood. The first intimation of the presence of this tumor is very often a swelling felt in the abdomen. Surgical removal and postoperative treatment will be necessary in these circumstances.

THE FUTURE

Children with Beckwith–Wiedemann syndrome should expect a normal life span, as long as malignancies do not occur. Any career is open to persons with this syndrome as long as mental abilities were not adversely affected by neonatal hypoglycemia.

Genetic counseling before pregnancy is advisable.

SELF-HELP GROUP

Beckwith–Wiedemann Support Network (BWSN)
3206 Braeburn Circle
Ann Arbor, MI 48108
734-973-0263 or 800-837-2976
email: a800bwsn@aol.com

Charcot–Marie–Tooth Disease

ALTERNATIVE NAMES

Peroneal muscular atrophy; CMT.

INCIDENCE

The incidence of Charcot–Marie–Tooth disease is undetermined, but it is estimated that around 130,000 Europeans are affected. There are a number of variations of Charcot–Marie–Tooth disease in which deafness and kidney disease are more apparent, and these variations are thought probably to be more common than Charcot–Marie–Tooth disease without these aspects. Boys and girls can be equally affected.

HISTORY

Charcot–Marie–Tooth disease is one of the most well-known of a group of familial diseases that have muscle weakness, mainly in the lower limbs, as their main symptom. The cause of this weakness is a degenerative process in the nerves supplying the muscles. There are a great many causes of this neuropathy, including other inherited diseases (for example, Friedrich ataxia), deficiency conditions such as diabetes and vitamin deficiencies, infectious conditions such as shingles, and the effects of various toxins (for example, botulism and certain drugs). Care must be taken that these causes are eliminated before a diagnosis of Charcot–Marie–Tooth disease is made.

In recent years, the genetic basis of the familial neuropathies has been established.

CAUSATION

Charcot–Marie–Tooth disease is most commonly inherited as an autosomal dominant, but it can also be inherited as an autosomal recessive characteristic. Prenatal diagnosis is possible with the dominant mode of inheritance. The severity of the symptoms can vary markedly in different individuals, with some aspects being more in evidence in some people than in others.

A few families have shown direct male-to-male inheritance. Recent reports have noted that a duplication of part of chromosome 17 seems to be responsible for Charcot–Marie–Tooth disease.

CHARACTERISTICS

Symptoms of Charcot–Marie–Tooth disease do not arise until the child is around 10 years old; they may appear later, even into middle age.

Legs and feet: Charcot–Marie–Tooth disease first shows itself in the lower limbs. The child's gait will become awkward, and he/she will not be able to keep up with his/her peers when speed is required. The muscles primarily affected are those running down the front of the lower leg. Thigh muscles are rarely involved in the muscle wasting that eventually becomes apparent in the lower leg as the legs characteristically assume a "stork-like" appearance. Ultimately, foot drop becomes obvious, with toes being dragged along as each step is taken. Fortunately, children with this condition rarely "go off their feet" altogether, and walking, although slow, can be maintained. Toes will later become fixed in a claw-like position caused by the wasting of muscle. Cramping and tingling sensations occur at a relatively early stage.

Fingers and arms: the upper limbs can be affected in a similar way to the legs and feet, but the effects on fingers and arms are usually milder in degree and the onset is later. The pathology of these effects is basically one of demyelination of the peripheral nerves, those supplying the muscles of the limbs, which gives rise to the characteristic symptoms of muscular weakness and eventually deformity.

Hearing: a sensorineural loss often becomes evident in later life. The first signs of deafness can occur in the teenage years, and by early middle age, the deafness is frequently severe.

Renal effects: nephritis can very occasionally be part of the symptomatology of Charcot–Marie–Tooth disease. If nephritis does occur, symptoms usually first begin to appear around the late twenties.

MANAGEMENT IMPLICATIONS

Mobility in childhood is the largest concern. In early years, mobility is frequently quite normal—the child walks, runs, and climbs along with his/her peers. In the school years, a child's difficulties with sports and other physical activities should alert care givers to possible problems. The child may complain of cramping pains in his/her legs. The diagnosis becomes obvious when muscle wasting and foot drop occurs. Children with Charcot–Marie–Tooth disease should not be pushed to take part in physical activities; they should instead be encouraged to pursue other interests that do not need too much physical exertion.

Advice and treatment from an orthopedic surgeon and a physical therapist regarding foot drop will help to prolong activity. Specially designed ankle–foot orthoses are valuable aids in combating foot drop. These aids can be conveniently worn under socks so that the child will not feel too different from his/her peers.

Hearing: the gradual loss of hearing that is a common feature of Charcot–Marie–Tooth disease must be monitored on a regular basis, and hearing aids should be fitted when hearing loss makes normal communication difficult.

THE FUTURE

Life expectancy is not limited by Charcot–Marie–Tooth disease. The main problems encountered will be ones of mobility and increasing deafness. Therefore, suitable careers must be chosen, bearing in mind the possible ongoing problems associated with this condition.

A watch must also be kept in early adult life for signs of renal problems that can occur at this time in persons suffering from this condition.

SELF-HELP GROUP

The Charcot–Marie–Tooth Association
601 Upland Avenue
Upland, PA 19015-2494
610-499-7486 or 800-606-CMTA
http://www.charcot-marie-tooth.org
email: CMTAssoc@aol.com

CHARGE Association

ALTERNATIVE NAMES

CHARGE syndrome; choanal atresia.

INCIDENCE

CHARGE association is a recently described condition, and only a few cases are recognized at present. "Association," rather than "syndrome," was thought to be a more appropriate term for this condition, as the cause has not been, as yet, isolated. The name, CHARGE, is an acronym of the main features seen. For a definite diagnosis to be made, at least two of the major features must be present. About twice as many boys as girls have so far been found to be affected.

HISTORY

In 1979, Dr. Hall first noticed the occurrence of other specific signs in association with the nasal defect of choanal atresia. (Choanal atresia is a life-threatening condition in which either one or both of the baby's nostrils are blocked by a bony or membranous defect. As all babies breathe entirely through their noses, it is vital that this type of blockage should be noted and treated urgently soon after birth.) In 1981, it was decided that CHARGE was an appropriate acronym for this set of symptoms.

In 1986, Dr. Davenport suggested that the condition should be termed a "syndrome" rather than an "association" of defects, as there was probably a common etiology for all the features seen. Either name is used now.

CAUSATION

Causation has not as yet been clarified. Most cases seem to be isolated ones, but both autosomal dominant and recessive modes of inheritance have been described. Family histories, as there are increasing numbers of babies found to be suffering from this condition, may help sort out this problem, although at present there are only a few recurrences in families. With prenatal ultrasound scanning, it is possible to note some of the abnormalities, such as heart defects.

CHARACTERISTICS

CHARGE is an acronym for Colomba of the eye; Heart disease; choanal Atresia; Retarded growth; Genital hypoplasia; Ear abnormalities.

Colomba of the eye is a defect in which parts of one, or a number of, the structures of the eye are missing. For example, there may be a "gap" in the iris or a similar defect in the retina or in other vital structures of the back of the eye. Defects in the latter structures are obviously of greater import than a defect in the iris, for they will directly affect vision. Eyelids can also be affected in a similar manner. Also, the whole eye may be smaller than normal. Effects on vision vary according to the type of defect present. About 80% of people with CHARGE association show this feature.

Heart defects are variable and range from complicated problems, such as tetralogy of Fallot, to a patent ductus arteriosus or a ventricular septal defect. Any baby born with choanal atresia must be examined carefully for signs of a heart defect because the two conditions occur together so frequently. The effects will depend on the type and the severity of the abnormality.

Choanal atresia was the first consistent sign to be noted in this collection of abnormalities. In some cases, only one nostril will be affected by the atresia, and, under these circumstances, the symptoms will be less severe. In fact, it may not be until the child has his/her first upper respiratory tract infection that the condition may be noticed, as there will be discharge of mucus from only one nostril and the other side of the nose will be unusually obstructed. In a severe bilateral case, it is vital that surgical treatment is undertaken early to repair the defect in order to prevent potentially lethal respiratory problems. With the less serious unilateral atresia, surgery can be elective, performed at a time when the child is more mature.

Retarded growth occurs in around 80% of babies with CHARGE association. Birth weight and length are usually normal, but by six months of age, growth has slowed so considerably that only the third percentile on standardized weight and height charts is reached. Subsequent growth continues along this lower line.

Genital hypoplasia of one kind or another is also found in children with CHARGE association. The most common form in boys is a small penis.

Ear abnormalities are not always present, and they can vary widely. Ears may have a characteristic triangular shape, or they may be extremely small. Hearing can also be affected, with deafness ranging from a mild loss to a profound one. Both conductive and sensorineural losses are seen.

These are the main features of CHARGE association, at least two of which must be present before a definite "label" can be attached to a particular case. There are also a number of other features that have been noted to be present in a high proportion of children with CHARGE association.

Learning difficulties are present in most children with this association; such problems can range from mild to severe.

Facial features including a small lower jaw and/or a cleft lip or palate are sometimes seen.

MANAGEMENT IMPLICATIONS

It is urgent that the **choanal atresia** is surgically corrected if the condition is bilateral. Following this surgery, respiratory function will be normal.

Heart defects must be looked for in all babies with choanal atresia and treated appropriately, if present.

If a **cleft lip or palate** is present, it will need surgical repair at some stage during the child's early years.

Vision must be checked in early childhood if any of the other features of CHARGE association are present. Although colomba of the iris is one of the more obvious features of the condition, it must be remembered that similar abnormalities can occur in other, less visible, parts of the eye.

Hearing problems should be fully investigated and treated as well as possible, if they exist. Hearing aids may be necessary for some children. If deafness is found to be present at an early age, intensive speech and language therapy will be necessary to ensure that the child does not miss out on the critical age for language acquisition.

Due to the frequency with which mental retardation occurs in association with the CHARGE condition, routine developmental checks must be carefully performed at the appropriate times. Following this monitoring, help can be given for any delays in specific, or general, areas of development.

Schooling, when the time comes, needs to be geared to the child's abilities; most children will manage adequately in mainstream schools, but some children may need extra help at specific times in different areas. The impact of hearing and visual problems as well as hospitalization, for cardiac or other problems, must also be remembered when schooling is being considered.

Genetic counseling, if further pregnancies are considered, is advisable.

THE FUTURE

Choanal atresia and heart problems are the two most serious features of CHARGE association. If these factors are adequately addressed, a normal life span is to be expected. Hearing, vision, and mild mental retardation can all make a difference when the choice of a career becomes paramount, and the effects of these problems must be considered.

SELF-HELP GROUP

CHARGE Syndrome Foundation, Inc.
2004 Parkade Boulevard
Columbia, MO 65202-3121
800-442-7604 or 573-499-4694
http://www.chargesyndrome.org
email: meg@chargesyndrome.org

Christmas Disease

ALTERNATIVE NAMES

Hemophilia B; factor 9 deficiency.

INCIDENCE

Christmas disease is one of the bleeding disorders of which hemophilia A is the most well known. For proper clotting of the blood following an injury, a number of "factors" are necessary. In Christmas disease the "factor" that is deficient is "factor 9." (Hemophilia A is deficient in "factor 8.")

The incidence of Christmas disease is 1 in every 50,000 live male births. Only boys are affected, due to the mode of inheritance. Christmas disease, and other bleeding disorders, are known worldwide and affect all races.

HISTORY

It was not until the early 1960s that specific treatment was available for diseases associated with bleeding problems. Until that time, much disability was suffered as a result of bleeding into the joints and soft tissues of the body following traumas of even a mild degree. With the advent of concentrates of the necessary clotting factors available for use after injury, this picture dramatically changed.

In recent years, many tragedies have occurred because a large proportion of hemophiliac patients contracted the HIV virus and AIDS from blood products contaminated with HIV. Heat treatment of the products used to treat hemophilia has now prevented the transmission of the HIV virus by factor concentrates.

CAUSATION

Christmas disease is inherited as an X-linked characteristic. The condition is passed down the female line from mothers, who suffer no ill-effects, to 50% of their sons.

Prenatal diagnosis can be made by fetoscopy. Measurement of the "factor 9" coagulation level, at birth, in a male baby who has a family history of a bleeding disorder will also give a diagnosis.

CHARACTERISTICS

As with hemophilia A, sufferers can be severely, moderately, or only mildly affected by Christmas disease. The degree of severity depends on the actual amount of factor 9 that is present in the blood. In severely affected boys, less than 1% of factor 9 will be normally active, while a mild sufferer can have as much as 20% of normally acting factor 9.

Boys with the severest manifestation of the condition will suffer **bleeding into the joints** following the slightest injury. For example, a bang on the knee or elbow that would hardly be noticed by other people will produce bleeding into the boy's joint with very obvious swelling and pain. Great care must be taken with children with hemophilia when they are learning to walk. Everyday tumbles onto knees in particular will produce painful bleeding episodes into these joints. Unless adequate treatment is given, these repeated, inevitable knocks of everyday life will cause damage to, and eventual destruction of, the joint. Great deformity, pain, and disability used to be the inevitable lot of persons with hemophilia (of whatever type).

Bleeding can also occur into the soft tissues of the body, and bruising is a frequent event following only mild trauma. In some instances, persons may confuse this easy bruising with signs of child abuse.

Minor surgical procedures, such as **tonsillectomy** or **dental extractions,** can lead to severe bleeding unless prophylactic treatment is given.

Infection with **hepatitis B** is a very real threat to boys with any of the bleeding disorders. This illness, characterized by general malaise, fever, lack of appetite, and jaundice, can lead to serious, potentially fatal, liver problems. Any boy with one of the bleeding disorders should be immunized against hepatitis B as soon as the diagnosis is made. Hepatitis C is also a concern. It usually causes a subclinical initial infection, but it can lead to cirrhosis and liver failure. No vaccine is currently available for it.

Treatment: the specific concentrate containing factor 9 must be used to treat hemorrhages as soon as possible after they have occurred. Parents can be given a supply of the concentrate to use promptly after their son has sustained an injury. This substance should also be given prophylactically before any surgical procedures are undertaken. Some boys may develop a type of immunity ("inhibitor") to their treatment. If that should happen, referral to a hematologist specializing in hemophilia should be made.

MANAGEMENT IMPLICATIONS

As with hemophilia A, a balance between overprotection and complete freedom must be decided upon by parents. The severity of their son's condition will obviously have a bearing on his activities. Contact sports and activities where there is a high potential for injury should be avoided. Mountaineering and canoeing are but two popular leisure activities that immediately come to mind as unsuitable for the boy with a bleeding disorder. The boy's interests should be channeled into less active, but equally interesting, hobbies.

Schooling in a mainstream setting should be possible. Teachers should be informed of their pupil's problems, and they should be aware of the action to be taken if an injury is sustained. To cope with the possibility of the boy's parents being unavailable if such an event should occur, the telephone number of the hematologist overseeing the boy's treatment should be made available at school. Education must be geared towards career choices that will be possible in the future for the boy with Christmas disease. Sedentary occupations with minimal physical content, and hence minimal injury potential, should be chosen.

Care should be taken when giving pain-relieving drugs to hemophiliac boys. Aspirin, and similar drugs that affect the function of platelets (important constituents in the blood intimately concerned with the clotting process), should be avoided.

THE FUTURE

With prompt treatment of hemorrhage, the possibility of long-term disability has vastly decreased, and boys with Christmas disease can live useful, fulfilling lives. Care will obviously have to be continued throughout life, and certain careers and leisure opportunities will not be open to these boys.

The only other possible problems connected with the disease are the possibilities of chronic hepatitis or infection with HIV. With immunization against hepatitis B and heat-treated blood products, these problems are reduced to a minimum.

SELF-HELP GROUP

World Federation of Hemophilia
1425 René Lévesque Boulevard West, Suite 1010
Montreal, Quebec H3G 1T7
Canada
514-875-7944
http://www.wfh.org
email: wfh@wfh.org

Cockayne Syndrome

INCIDENCE

Cockayne syndrome is very rare, but it is well documented in the literature. The syndrome has been reported from the USA, Japan, and Europe. Boys and girls are equally affected. There is a subgroup known as Cockayne syndrome type 2, in which the age of onset is much earlier. Boys are three times as likely to be affected as girls with this subgroup.

CAUSATION

Cockayne syndrome is inherited as an autosomal recessive condition. It is thought that an enzyme defect is the basic fault. The deficient enzyme, or enzymes, are those responsible for the repair of cells following exposure to sunlight. The relationship between these effects and the other neurological problems of the syndrome are unclear at present.

Amniocentesis at 16 weeks can determine the syndrome prenatally.

CHARACTERISTICS

The baby with Cockayne syndrome is normal at birth. All aspects of growth and development appear to be proceeding normally until the child is between 6 and 12 months of age. The following characteristics then make their appearance:

Growth is drastically reduced after the initial period of normal growth. All routine measurements—height, weight, and head circumference—lag when plotted on the normal growth charts. Severe dwarfism is the final result. Subcutaneous fat and tissue are also lost, resulting in a wizened appearance, rather like that seen in extreme old age. By the time the child is four years old, this appearance is very obvious.

Mental retardation: the restriction in physical growth is accompanied by a decline in mental abilities, which, regrettably, is progressive. The actual brain tissue atrophies, and demyelination of all nerves is seen. These factors account for the progressive loss of skills.

Skin: the majority of children with Cockayne syndrome have a severe sensitivity to the sun. A scaly, red rash develops after only minimal exposure to sunlight. This rash is followed by crusting and eventually scarring, together with excessive pigmentation of the affected areas.

These effects are a direct result of the skin's failure to repair damaged cells, which is in turn is due to the enzyme abnormality.

Eyes: cataracts and retinal atrophy frequently occur with increasing age, making a blindness a very real possibility.

Ears: sensorineural deafness is also common.

MANAGEMENT IMPLICATIONS

Mental retardation: the severe progressive loss of skills, both mental and physical, seen in a child with Cockayne syndrome is devastating for the parents. Continuing, sensitive counseling is necessary to help parents through this time. The child will eventually need full-time care. Incontinence, mobility difficulties, and visual and auditory defects all add to the handicap.

Skin: great care must be taken to avoid exposure to sunlight. Protective clothing, including hats with brims to protect the face, as well as strict avoidance of really bright sunlight must be the order of the day. Protective clothing needs to be worn even on overcast days. High SPF sunscreen can also be applied.

Vision and hearing: deficits in the special senses will need to be checked regularly. Little can be done to prevent the progressive losses of sight and hearing, but care givers can remember the gradual loss of those methods of communication and attempt to use other methods of contact with the progressively handicapped child.

THE FUTURE

Many children with Cockayne syndrome die in early childhood, but some reach the late teens. Handicap becomes profound, and full-time care will be needed.

SELF-HELP GROUP

Share and Care Cockayne Syndrome Network
P.O. Box 552
Stanleytown, VA 24168
540-629-2369

Coffin–Lowry Syndrome

ALTERNATIVE NAME

Coffin syndrome.

INCIDENCE

Coffin–Lowry syndrome was thought to be a rare syndrome, but it now appears to be more common than the number of published cases suggests. Both boys and girls can be affected, and the syndrome has been reported in many countries throughout the world.

HISTORY

The syndrome was described by Dr. Coffin in 1966 and by Dr. Lowry in 1971.

CAUSATION

Coffin–Lowry syndrome is an X-linked recessive condition. Family studies have shown inheritance to be strongly linked through the female line. Sporadic cases due to new mutations are also thought to occur frequently.

CHARACTERISTICS

Mental retardation: this aspect of Coffin–Lowry syndrome appears to be worse in boys than in girls. Most boys with the condition are severely retarded. Girls can be similarly affected, but they more frequently have only mild retardation or have completely normal intellectual function.

Short stature is not excessive, but most children with Coffin–Lowry syndrome grow along the third percentile of the growth charts for height. Final height is rarely more than 5 feet. During adolescence, scoliosis and kyphosis commonly occur, which adds to the apparent shortness of stature. Puberty occurs at the usual time.

Facial features: foreheads are square with widely set apart eyes and a short nose. The mouth tends to be large with a full lower lip and a small lower jaw. Features often become coarsened with age.

Fingers have a very characteristic shape, being both puffy and tapering toward the tips. An excess of soft tissue accounts for the puffy appearance. Fingers are also often hyperextendible due to laxity of the ligaments surrounding the joints. (In some children, this laxity also extends to other joints of the body.)

Deafness can be a problem, although it is by no means inevitable.

Seizures can occur, but, again, not every child with Coffin–Lowry syndrome will be affected in this way.

MANAGEMENT IMPLICATIONS

Learning difficulties: the management of this aspect of Coffin–Lowry syndrome will depend on the degree of handicap found in the individual child. Serial developmental testing throughout childhood is important so educational facilities can be tailored to ensure that the child's full potential is reached.

Boys with this syndrome rarely achieve normal speech. Speech therapy can help evaluate the level of language attained and to assist with greater fluency and language acquisition.

Scoliosis and/or **kyphosis:** in adolescence, a close watch for these vertebral abnormalities is necessary. Referral for an orthopedic surgeon's opinion, and possible treatment, is advisable for all but the mildest of abnormalities. The chest deformity that can result from the vertebral problems can give rise to respiratory problems. Early orthopedic intervention can largely prevent this complication, however.

Deafness should be remembered as a possibility in children with Coffin–Lowry syndrome. Hearing should be tested at regular intervals.

Seizures must be controlled with appropriate anticonvulsants.

THE FUTURE

Life expectancy appears to be limited to around 40 years. Death usually occurs from cardiac or respiratory problems, often as a result of the spinal defects so commonly seen.

Boys will need special educational facilities. Girls, too, may require special teaching, but girls frequently have normal intellectual abilities and can successfully pursue normal schooling and careers.

SELF-HELP GROUP

Coffin–Lowry Syndrome Foundation (CLSF)
Mary Hoffman
3045 255th Avenue S.E.
Issaquah, WA 98029
425-427-0939
http://www.freeyellow.com/members3/clsf/index/html
email: CLSFoundation@yahoo.com

Cohen Syndrome

Pepper syndrome

INCIDENCE

This is a rare syndrome, with both boys and girls being affected. It has been suggested that the condition is more common in Ashkenazi Jewish populations.

This syndrome bears some similarities to both Prader–Willi and Laurence–Moon syndromes. For correct diagnosis of Cohen syndrome, five of the specific characteristics are considered necessary to be present, but the effects of the disorder can vary greatly from individual to individual.

CAUSATION

Cohen syndrome is though to be autosomally inherited, and the gene has been mapped to chromosome 8. Prenatal diagnosis has not, as yet, been reported, but it may be possible in the future.

CHARACTERISTICS

Obesity is an almost universal feature in children with Cohen syndrome. As with Prader–Willi syndrome, in which children also have a weight problem, obesity can be difficult to control.

Small jaws are a further common feature of Cohen syndrome. Both upper and lower jaws can be affected, or only one jaw can have this feature. In many children with this condition, the top two incisor teeth are very prominent and overlap the bottom incisors. This feature can lead to an unusual "bite" and give rise to chewing difficulties. It can also make for a very characteristic facial appearance. Along with the small mouth, the palate is high and arched.

Small, narrow hands and feet and a **short stature** are all part of the general slow growth. Flat feet with a tendency to knock-knees, together with an excessive hollowing of the lower back, are other commonly found skeletal features.

Joints can be overly extendable so that fingers and arms can more easily than usual be contorted into unusual postures. Such postures are made especially easy by the general lack of muscle tone that is frequently also present.

Eye abnormalities can include myopia, a lazy eye, and occasionally other problems affecting the retina.

Learning difficulties are relatively common, but in some children they are present to only a mild degree.

Cohen syndrome has a number of features that, in isolation, can be thought to be mild deviations from what is considered normal. It is when a number of these characteristics are present together that a firm diagnosis of the syndrome can be made.

MANAGEMENT IMPLICATIONS

Control of **obesity** from an early age is important. Advice from a dietitian is valuable and can set good eating patterns for life. Overweight children can suffer considerably from teasing during school years; they can have difficulty in enjoying physical activities; and, of course, obesity has implications for a healthy later life. Therefore, if the child's weight can be controlled in the preschool years, much heartache will be avoided later.

Regular **dental checks** are vitally important. Over-crowding of teeth readily occurs because of the small size of the jaws. Orthodontic treatment of the unusual "bite" can be necessary when the second set of teeth appear. Tooth enamel can also be less than perfect in children with Cohen syndrome, causing decay to occur more readily than is normal.

Orthopedic treatment is sometimes necessary to correct joint abnormalities that can give rise to mobility problems.

Visual problems, such as myopia and lazy eye, will need ophthalmic advice and treatment. The more serious potential retinal problems will require regular checks.

Learning difficulties or earlier developmental delays in attaining the normal milestones will need multidisciplinary assessment. Strengths should be fostered, and any areas of special difficulty will need specialized help to minimize the effects. If the learning difficulty hinders the child from keeping up with peers at school, assistance should be organized. Assessments must be ongoing throughout the learning years and followed by help and advice for suitable career options.

THE FUTURE

The future will depend upon which features of Cohen syndrome are most prevalent in the individual child. None of the characteristics are life-threatening, and a normal life span is usual. Careers will need to be geared to the person's physical and intellectual abilities, but a fully independent life style is the general rule.

SELF-HELP GROUPS

There are no known self-help groups in the United States, but further information may be obtained from:

National Organization for Rare Disorders, Inc. (NORD)
P.O. Box 8923
New Fairfield, CT 06812-8923
203-746-6518 or 800-999-6673
http://www.nord-rdb.com/~orphan
email: orphan@nord-rdb.com

Cohen Syndrome Support Group
7 Woods Court
Brackley, Northants NN13- 6HP
United Kingdom
012-80-704515

Congenital Central Hypoventilation Syndrome

ALTERNATIVE NAME

Ondine's curse.

INCIDENCE

Congenital central hypoventilation syndrome is a rare condition, which may be congenital or follow an acquired viral encephalitis. Both boys and girls can be affected. Swift diagnosis is extremely important so that life saving treatment can be given.

CAUSATION

There is no known definitive genetic cause for this syndrome, but because the basic cause is a failure of the autonomic system to control respiration (due to a probable chemoreceptor fault), it is likely that there is a genetic fault.

It is probable that the condition occurs sporadically and that there is little likelihood that the condition will recur in later pregnancies, although some authorities have suggested an autosomal recessive inheritance with incomplete penetrance.

There can at times, however, be a link with specific gut mobility disorders—particularly Hirschsprung disease. (See below.)

There is no prenatal diagnosis possible.

CHARACTERISTICS

Breathing during sleep is insufficient in this condition. This problem is especially evident during periods of "quiet" sleep. In REM (rapid eye movement) sleep, breathing can be almost normal.

Cyanosis—blue coloration of the skin due to lack of oxygenation of the tissues—is frequently the first noticeable sign of the syndrome, starting soon after birth. Parents may also initially become aware that something is wrong by observing periods of apnea (lack of any breathing movements) when their baby is asleep.

Seizures during sleep will occasionally be the first signs of the syndrome. These seizures are due to lack of oxygen to the brain.

Urine production, which is usually reduced during the night (due to the secretion of a specific antidiuretic hormone [ADH]), can be reversed, giving rise to wet beds or, in the older child, frequent waking to urinate.

Body temperature control may be affected, so that extremes of both heat and cold are poorly tolerated. **Hearing** problems have also been reported.

Hirschsprung disease is a gut mobility condition that affects the passage of food through the lower part of the large bowel. It is thought that around 18% of children with congenital central ventilation syndrome will also have this condition.

Hirschsprung disease affects the ability of the autonomic nervous system to control a segment of the lower bowel. The peristaltic waves of alternating contraction and relaxation that pass through the whole intestine and force the food onward are absent in the affected part of the gut. The result is severe constipation beginning in the neonatal period, with large masses of feces being held in the grossly distended lower part of the colon just above the rectum.

X-ray studies show the distended bowel, and on physical examination, the blockage can be felt by the examining finger. Biopsy of a part of the lower bowel will clinch the diagnosis.

Severe enterocolitis, which shows itself by diarrhea and circulatory collapse, can be a complication of this disease. This complication can be rapidly fatal unless urgent medical treatment is available.

(It must be stressed that this condition does not occur in all children with congenital central ventilation syndrome, but the possibility needs to be remembered. Hirschsprung disease can also be present as a clinical entity on its own.)

MANAGEMENT IMPLICATIONS

Respiratory support by positive pressure ventilation is necessary during sleep and may be needed at other times during the day when respiration is insufficient. (Insufficient respiration sometimes occurs when a child is concentrating deeply on a specific task or is suffering from some intercurrent infection.) It is more usual, however, for respiratory support to be only needed during night-time sleep. The child will likely continue to need this support over the long term, as the condition does not appear to improve spontaneously.

It is important that respiratory infections in children with this syndrome are treated immediately and adequately. Further difficulties in breathing, due to the infection, can quickly decompensate the already compromised respiration.

Seizures will usually cease once the respiratory problems have been adequately treated, but anticonvulsant drugs may be necessary in some instances.

Enuresis should be dealt with sympathetically if it occurs. Usual toilet training methods can prove difficult to implement due to the failure of the usual hormonal control of night-time urination. Waking the child at intervals is a possible solution.

Children with this condition should avoid **extremes of temperature.** Cooling on very hot days or under hot conditions and keeping warm in cold weather need to be priorities.

Hearing needs to be checked regularly, and any parental doubts regarding possible deafness should be noted and acted upon.

Surgery is necessary to correct the bowel abnormality associated with **Hirschsprung disease.**

THE FUTURE

The future will, of course, depend upon the severity of the condition. In the most severe cases, respiratory support may be needed throughout the day, but the majority of children will only need support at night or when asleep during the day.

SELF-HELP GROUP

Congenital Central Hypoventilation Syndrome (CCHS) Family Support
  Network
71 Maple Street
Oneonta, NY 13820
607-432-8872
email: VanderlaanM@Hartwick.edu

Cornelia De Lange Syndrome

ALTERNATIVE NAMES

De Lange syndrome; Brachmannde Lange syndrome; Amsterdam dwarfism.

INCIDENCE

It is estimated that 1 in every 10,000 babies born alive will be affected by this syndrome. Boys and girls are equally affected.

HISTORY

Cornelia de Lange syndrome was first published as a clinical entity in 1933. Dr. Brachmann had previously also described the condition in 1916.

CAUSATION

The cause of this serious condition still remains a mystery. Some children with Cornelia de Lange syndrome have chromosomal abnormalities, but these are not consistently confined to one chromosome. Two research programs—one in the UK, and one in the USA—are currently in progress to determine the etiology of this syndrome.

Some of the specific abnormalities associated with the syndrome can be detected on ultrasound. Apart from ultrasound, there is no prenatal diagnostic test available at present. Cornelia de Lange syndrome is obvious at birth.

CHARACTERISTICS

Learning disability is inevitably present in Cornelia de Lange syndrome, but the disability can vary in degree from mild to severe handicap. All aspects of development are delayed. Speech is especially late, and it may be absent altogether. Children with this condition, however, often have relatively good motor and spatial skills. Some children with Cornelia de Lange syndrome show certain autistic features such as limited social contact abilities and repetitive or obsessive routines. Unusual, hyperactive behavior is common, with self mutilation on occasions being a particularly worrying aspect.

Skeletal system: birth weight is frequently low despite a full-term pregnancy. Children are short and have a reduced head circumference (microcephaly). Noses are small and tip-tilted so that nostrils are very obvious.

Arms: there are often severe abnormalities ranging from tiny hands with a single palmar crease to, in some cases, partial absence of the upper limbs.

Legs are generally normal and fully formed, but there is often webbing of the second and third toes.

Babies with Cornelia de Lange syndrome are floppy at birth, and they tend to remain **hypotonic** throughout their lives.

Heart defects commonly occur, and they may be of any type—no specific abnormality is typical.

Seizures occur in many children with Cornelia de Lange syndrome.

Excess hair is frequently seen all over the body. The eyebrows are especially bushy and often meet in the mid-line over the bridge of the nose.

Infections of all kinds can cause problems throughout life, as Cornelia de Lange children seem to have a very much reduced resistance to all types.

MANAGEMENT IMPLICATIONS

During infancy, **feeding** and **breathing** problems are common, due both to the low birth weight and to the microcephaly. Babies will frequently need to be in an incubator and fed by a nasogastric tube for the first few weeks of life.

Seizures need to be treated with anticonvulsant drugs. Several of these drugs, or combinations of drugs, may need to be tried before satisfactory control is achieved.

Infections will need aggressive treatment with antibiotics throughout life, due to the child's increased susceptibility to all types of everyday infections.

Any **heart defect** will need assessment, regular monitoring, and/or treatment with drugs or surgery as necessary.

Intellectual abilities will also need to be carefully and regularly assessed. It has been found that children with Cornelia de Lange syndrome respond very readily to care and stimulation of all kinds. All babies need to be spoken to on a regular basis from an early age. Speech and other stimuli will ensure that each child reaches his or her full genetic potential. This aspect of childcare is especially important if there is any degree of learning disability.

Behavioral modification techniques can be helpful in reducing difficult behavior.

Schooling: the child will require "special needs" placement as appropriate locally. Children with Cornelia de Lange syndrome will thrive best in a warm, loving family environment with specialized teaching to maximize the motor and spatial skills.

Children with severe **upper limb deformities** will need help from a rehabilitation center that specializes in artificial limbs. Special equipment may be necessary for some children to maximize abilities.

THE FUTURE

An independent lifestyle is only possible for those individuals who are mildly affected. Few people with this syndrome reach old age. Their increased susceptibility to infection and the long-term consequences of possible heart defects make for serious life-threatening problems.

SELF-HELP GROUP

Cornelia de Lange Syndrome Foundation
302 West Main Street, #100
Avon, CT 06001
860-676-8166 or 800-753-CDLS
http://cdlsoutreach.org
email: cdlsintl@iconn.net

Cri Du Chat Syndrome

ALTERNATIVE NAMES

Chromosome 5 short-arm deletion; 5p–syndrome; Lejeune syndrome.

INCIDENCE

It is thought that up to one percent of all profoundly retarded children suffer from this syndrome. Until genetic studies became available, this syndrome was not classified, although the very typical cry during infancy had been noted.

The exact incidence is not known, but it is probably about 1 in 20,000 births. The sexes appear to be affected equally, although it has been suggested that cri du chat syndrome is more common in girls.

HISTORY

Professor Lejeune fully documented this syndrome in the 1960s.

CAUSATION

Cri du chat syndrome is a chromosomal disorder. The chromosome affected is chromosome 5; the short arm of this chromosome is deleted in children affected by this syndrome. Most cases arise as a new mutation, although a balanced translocation may be present in one or other of the parents. Under this latter circumstance, there is an increased risk of recurrence in a future pregnancy. Neither parent's age appears to have any bearing on the advent of the syndrome.

Prenatal diagnosis can be made by chorionic villus sampling at 9 to 12 weeks of pregnancy, and later (16 weeks) by amniocentesis.

CHARACTERISTICS

A **weak, high-pitched cry** is the most obvious characteristic of cri du chat syndrome. This cry is very like that of a kitten—hence the name of the syndrome. The reason for this typical cry is the relatively small size of the larynx. As this structure enlarges with growth, the unusual cat-like cry is lost.

Short stature: birth weight of babies with cri du chat syndrome is usually on the low side of average. Throughout life, children with this syndrome are small, rarely growing to a height above that measured on the third percentile of the standard growth charts.

Facial characteristics: ninety-eight percent of cri du chat children are microcephalic. Head circumference is small at birth and continues to grow only slowly. Children with this syndrome have round faces with a downward slant to the eyes, which are widely set apart. There is often also a divergent lazy eye present.

Congenital heart disease is a relatively common occurrence in children with cri du chat syndrome. Around 30% of the affected children have this problem, the defect most usually being a patent ductus arteriosus. The murmur of this abnormality can usually be heard at birth. Symptoms of heart disease will depend on severity of the defect.

Learning disability is always severe; there are no reports of children with an IQ higher than 35. Evidence of this retardation can be suspected in the early months of life when the milestones of smiling, following objects visually, and later reaching out for toys are absent or much delayed. As development proceeds, the retardation, regrettably, becomes more and more obvious.

Poor muscle tone: the baby with cri du chat syndrome is floppy at birth and can experience severe breathing difficulties. Head control is slow in being attained, and movements are restricted. Most adults with the condition have poor muscle development.

Speech: Language development is frequently delayed—some children being able to make their needs known by speech while others find gestures and/or sign language an easier method of communication.

MANAGEMENT IMPLICATIONS

During infancy, there are severe **respiratory** and **feeding** difficulties. These problems are due both to the small size of the larynx and associated structures and to the general floppiness of the baby. The baby may initially need to be in an incubator to promote adequate respiration. Tube feeding may also be necessary for proper nutrition. Even if the baby can suck adequately, feeding is very slow, which in turn exhausts the hypotonic baby. Respiratory problems improve with the growth in size of the respiratory passages over the succeeding months.

Congenital heart disease may require surgical repair. (Whether or not surgery is necessary depends on the site and size of the defect, as well as the effects of the defect on the baby's cardiac function.) Obviously, the baby's general condition will need to be carefully assessed, and steps to improve both nutritional and respiratory functions must be taken before any surgery is contemplated.

Learning disability: it has been specifically noted that early and frequent stimulation of the baby with cri du chat syndrome is beneficial. Therefore, verbal stimulation—talking continually to the baby while attending to his/her needs—as well as other auditory and visual stimuli are important in developing all possible mental abilities. Few children with this syndrome develop normal communication skills, but, with sufficient, appropriate stimuli, some responses and feedback from the child can be gained—albeit at a very primitive level.

Children with cri du chat syndrome, like all other children, are happiest and reach their maximum potential if they can be brought up in the warmth and security of their own homes, or alternatively in a secure, stable environment with plenty of one-on-one contact.

Walking skills are usually attained late. This delay is due both to the hypotonia seen in infancy and to the degree of mental retardation. Structured exercise from a physical therapist may help the child to walk and will aid muscle development.

Lazy eye, if present, may need correction for cosmetic reasons and also to ensure that maximum visual input can be received—the latter is even more important for a handicapped child than for a child who can more readily adapt. Amblyopia can develop all too quickly in an untreated lazy eye.

THE FUTURE

The child with severe symptoms due to cri du chat syndrome will have difficulty in leading an independent life. Others, with only moderate learning difficulties, can manage much of their own self care. Life span is limited, mainly due to respiratory and/or cardiac problems, but many children survive into adulthood. The oldest recorded adult with cri du chat syndrome is 56 years of age.

SELF-HELP GROUP

5p– Society
7108 Katella Avenue, #502
Stanton, CA 90680
714-901-1544 or 888-970-0777
http://www.fivepminus.org
email: fivepminus@aol.com

Crouzon Syndrome

ALTERNATIVE NAME

Craniofacial dystosis.

INCIDENCE

The exact incidence of Crouzon syndrome is unknown, but it is a rare condition. However the incidence of similar conditions that also have abnormalities of the head and face are not uncommon. It has been estimated that 1 in every 2,000 children will have such abnormalities. There are many syndromes associated with this type of disfigurement: for example, Pfeiffer syndrome, Apert syndrome (see elsewhere in the text), and Carpenter syndrome. Boys and girls are affected in equal numbers.

The condition can be recognized at birth by the unusual facial features, and it can be confirmed by X-ray examination.

No prenatal diagnosis is available at present.

CAUSATION

Crouzon syndrome can be inherited as an autosomal dominant condition. In these circumstances, there is a wide variety in the physical expression of the disease—some cases being more severe than others.

In around 50% of cases, however, the condition appears as a fresh mutation. Some authorities consider these sporadic occurrences of Crouzon syndrome to be associated with advanced paternal age.

CHARACTERISTICS

The basic defect occurring in Crouzon syndrome is a premature fusion of the bones of the skull. The bones of a baby's skull are normally joined together by fibrous tissue in specific places, known as "sutures." This comparatively loose connection of the bones of the skull allows for enlargement of the underlying brain during the early growing years, and it also allows for "molding" of the baby's head as it passes down the birth canal. In Crouzon syndrome, the early closure of these sutures results in the specific features seen in the head and faces of babies with this condition.

The **head** is small—a fact directly due to the early closure of the bones of the skull. On feeling the baby's head, there will be no normal fontanelles—instead, the bones of the head are part of one continuous structure. (The anterior and posterior fontanelles on the baby's head are two gaps in the skull where the brain is covered only by strong fibrous tissue. These fontanelles normally are closed by around 18 months of age.) The foreheads of these babies are usually high and can bulge forward.

A **cleft palate** may be present. In the most severe cases, under-development of the external meatus of the ear can occur.

On X-ray examination, the **paranasal sinuses** are also seen to be small.

Facial features: Probably the most striking facial feature of the baby with Crouzon syndrome is the shallow orbit containing the eyes. This feature has the effect of causing the eyes to protrude. There may also be a markedly divergent lazy eye and/or nystagmus. The optic nerve may also be damaged due to the bony abnormalities. This damage can result in optic atrophy with advancing blindness.

The nose is characteristically beaked, and the septum—dividing the two sides of the nose—can be deviated to one side, causing obstruction to normal nasal breathing.

Teeth, when they erupt, are often overcrowded and malformed. This problem is due, in part, to the malformation of the jaw. The upper jaw tends to be smaller than normal. This feature, combined with a normal sized lower jaw, tends to give the baby a pugnacious appearance.

Learning disability is regretfully a common finding in children with Crouzon syndrome.

A common complication of this condition is **increased cranial pressure,** which is a direct result of the premature closure of the bones of the skull.

The above description is of the most severely affected child. Due to the wide variation in the expressivity of the condition, less severely affected children are seen. In some cases, it is only when the skull is X-rayed that the syndrome is diagnosed.

MANAGEMENT IMPLICATIONS

In the early days of life, **breathing** may be a problem if the nose is severely affected. (All newborn babies breathe solely through their noses, so any problems with this feature can have serious consequences.)

Neurosurgical intervention will be urgently needed if signs of **raised intracranial pressure** occur. Signs of raised pressure will be vomiting, irritability, and/or seizures. In an older child, headaches can occur or vision can become blurred. This type of surgery is usually needed during the first three months of life.

Other surgical techniques may be necessary later in life to correct unusual **facial features.**

Regular **developmental checks** will need to be done to asssess progress in all the areas of development. In conjunction with developmental examinations, extra checks on vision and hearing will need to be done regularly to identify any deterioration in these special senses.

Schooling will need to be geared to each individual child's specific needs, taking into account the degree of mental ability, vision, and hearing. Again, close liaison between education and health authorities is vital.

THE FUTURE

Life expectancy is normal for a child with Crouzon syndrome. The quality of life will depend very much on the severity of the condition as it affects each individual.

SELF-HELP GROUPS

Crouzon Support Network
P.O. Box 1272
Edmonds, WA 98020
425-672-1697
http://www.crouzon.org

Children's Craniofacial Association
P.O. Box 280297
Dallas, TX 75228
972-994-9902 or 800-535-3643
email: DNKM90A@prodigy.com

Cystic Fibrosis

ALTERNATIVE NAMES

Cystic fibrosis of pancreas; mucoviscoidosis. (Both these names are rarely used these days, but they may be found in old articles.)

INCIDENCE

Cystic fibrosis is very common, especially among persons of Northern European descent. African and Asian populations rarely suffer from this condition.

The incidence in the affected white populations is as high as 1 birth in every 2,000 to 2,500. Both boys and girls can be affected.

CAUSATION

Cystic fibrosis is inherited as an autosomal recessive. About 1 in 20 to 1 in 25 people carry the abnormal gene in the populations affected by the disease. Carriers have no symptoms of cystic fibrosis, but a baby conceived by two carriers of the condition will show the typical characteristics of cystic fibrosis.

There can be several genes that show mutations causing cystic fibrosis. It is thought that the degree of severity suffered depends on which gene disorder is present. Active research is continuing into this possibility, as well as many other aspects of cystic fibrosis. The basic fault occurring as a result of these altered genes is in the protein CFTR. This protein is responsible for the passage of salt ions across the membranes of cells in the body. As a result of this fault, sticky mucus is produced in various organs. The lungs and pancreas are mainly involved, but the liver and sweat glands also show changes. It is the effects of this excess of sticky mucus that gives rise to the problems seen in cystic fibrosis, together with the resultant subsequent damage to many organs in the body.

Prenatal diagnosis is possible by chorionic villus sampling and/or amniocentesis. If a person is related to affected individuals, that person can be tested for carrier status.

CHARACTERISTICS

One of the very first signs that a baby has cystic fibrosis can appear in the very early days of life. Obstruction of the bowel can occur by the buildup of sticky meconium—that waste product in the baby's bowel normally passed soon after birth. This condition is known as **meconium ileus.** Around 5 to 10% of babies with cystic fibrosis have this early complication of the disorder.

Lungs are the organs most seriously affected by cystic fibrosis. Buildup of sticky mucus in the respiratory passages (nose and sinuses as well as lungs) results in frequent and severe respiratory infections from an early age. These repeated infections will eventually cause permanent damage to the lungs. Treatment is by antibiotics for each bout of infection, but difficult-to-treat infections, such as those caused by the Pseudomonas bacteria, unfortunately become more common as the child matures. A vaccine against this particular form of infection is currently being evaluated.

The mainstay of treatment for the lung problems of cystic fibrosis, as well as appropriate antibiotic therapy, is regular physical therapy, on a three-times-a-day basis. Through postural drainage, the child is able to cough up some of the sticky mucus that is continually being accumulated in his/her lungs. Parents become very adept at giving their child this form of physical therapy, but it can become an enormous burden to carry out this time-consuming and demanding (for both parent and child) treatment three times every day—Saturdays, Sundays, holidays, and school days. In recent years, heart-lung transplants have been carried out on children with severe cystic fibrosis with a good deal of success.

In addition to the symptoms in the respiratory tract, the **digestive system** is also affected. The deficiency of specific enzymes from the pancreas gives rise to digestive problems, as the enzyme lack causes food to be inadequately digested and absorbed. Within a few months, the baby will not be thriving as well as could be expected. Weight gain is slow, and anemia due to specific malabsorption of iron-containing foods can result if the diagnosis is not made and appropriate treatment given. Treatment consists of regular medication with pancreatic enzyme-replacement products. With this drug regimen and a highly nutritious diet (for which specialized advice from a dietitian is necessary in the early days), the child will start to gain weight. Extra salt will also need to be given, as salt is lost in excess through the sweat glands in children with cystic fibrosis. This problem is especially important to remember in hot weather. Salt depletion can give rise to serious heat prostration.

Sweat glands in cystic fibrosis children are involved in the generalized disorder of many glands of the body. The excess salt that is excreted by these glands, found all over the body, is the basis for the conclusive diagnostic test for cystic fibrosis. Excess sweat, induced by a specialized technique, is analyzed. Cystic fibrosis sufferers have levels of salt loss through these glands that are up to twice as high as normal levels.

The **liver,** the largest gland in the body and involved in many aspects of metabolism, can be affected by blockage of ducts with sticky mucus. In a few children, this vital organ can become damaged by the blockage.

Prolapse of the rectum (protrusion of part of the lower bowel at the anus) is a further clue to the diagnosis of cystic fibrosis. The prolapse occurs only in around 5 to 10% of children with cystic fibrosis, but for these children, repeated episodes of this problem may occur. This problem may seem minor when compared with the serious effects in the lungs and digestive system, but it is nevertheless a worrying one for parents. Gentle replacement of the bowel is all that is necessary.

Cystic fibrosis is a serious, life-threatening disease, but it is being extensively researched. Hopefully, within a decade, gene therapy will be the answer to many of the problems.

MANAGEMENT IMPLICATIONS

Lung problems are the most serious aspect of cystic fibrosis. Frequent infections needing urgent and prolonged antibiotic treatment will occur. Fighting these infections, which also cause loss of appetite, will add to the problems of normal growth and weight gain, while the necessary ongoing physical therapy eats into the daily lives of both parents and children.

When **school** days arrive, the demands of infections and physical therapy make for difficulties. When frequent absences with respiratory infection are a fact of life, keeping up with schoolwork can cause problems. Sympathetic help, with suitable work sent home and extra help at school when the child is well, can do much to help and encourage families with children with cystic fibrosis. Long hospital admissions are often necessary for many children with cystic fibrosis. Liaison with the child's school can help to keep the child interested and also prevent him/her from missing large sections of work.

Physical therapy in the middle of the school day can be a problem. Many and varied are the ways of overcoming this difficulty, depending on local facilities. In an ideal situation, nursing or physical therapy help can be made available for a mid-day physical therapy session. During the elementary-school years, parents can be made welcome in school to fulfill this task if the child is not able to go home for lunch. Sufficient space, of course, must also be made available in which to do the physical therapy—often a problem for many schools. Children can learn the proper positions for their own postural drainage at a surprisingly early age. A controlled exercise program is a vital part of the physical therapy program, and parents and other care givers should encourage the child to continue with these activities. Swimming is excellent therapy. Antibiotic treatment can be continued in school for the older cystic fibrosis child if teachers are willing to supervise medication. Older children needing intravenous antibiotic treatment can be fitted with a special device so that injections can continue while the children are attending school. Under these circumstances, the child concerned must be capable and willing to undertake this part of his/her own treatment.

Diet is important in the management of children with cystic fibrosis. Today's thinking on this aspect of treatment emphasizes a high-calorie diet in order to maintain growth. The continual help of a dietitian is vital to ensure that the best combination of suitable foods is given. School meals must be monitored, and teachers should be informed of the specific needs of their pupil with cystic fibrosis. Frequent oily, bulky, and foul-smelling stools can be a difficult problem, and they may indicate that the intake of fat in the diet needs to be reduced. To help with this offensive odor at home and at school, there are several commercially available deodorizers that are very effective.

Recreation is as important for the child with cystic fibrosis as it is for anyone else, but it must be geared to the child's needs. Many children with cystic fibrosis pursue active sports, but these activities must be monitored carefully so as not to further damage lung capacity. (This observation also applies, of course, to physical education in school.) When taking a cystic fibrosis child to a hot climate, adequate salt replacement must be borne in mind.

Sexual development is often delayed in children with cystic fibrosis, often by as much as two years.

THE FUTURE

The future depends very much on the severity of the disease. Many children do not survive beyond their early twenties, but with several treatment changes in view, this outlook seems set to improve within the foreseeable future: antibiotic treatment is improving all the time; heart-lung transplants are proving successful in prolonging life for severely affected children; and gene therapy, in which the damaged gene is replaced by a normal one, is being actively researched. The latter will doubtless come to fruition within the foreseeable future.

SELF-HELP GROUPS

Cystic Fibrosis Foundation
6931 Arlington Road
Bethesda, MD 20814
301-951-4422 or 800-344-4823
http://www.cff.org
email: info@cff.org

Cystic Fibrosis Alliance
P.O. Box 4213
Ft. Lauderdale, FL 33338
305-463-4440

Down Syndrome

ALTERNATIVE NAMES

Trisomy 21; mongolism (obsolete).

INCIDENCE

Down syndrome is the most well known chromosomal abnormality. The overall incidence in Caucasian, Japanese, and African American populations is between 1 in every 660 births and 1 in every 800 births. The incidence of Down syndrome is very dependent on the age of the mother. The risk rises sharply when the mother is older than 35 years old. Both boys and girls can be affected by Down syndrome.

HISTORY

Down syndrome has been recognized for many years. In the early part of the twentieth century, Dr. Langdon Down specifically and accurately described all the features associated with the condition.

CAUSATION

Down syndrome is caused by a chromosomal abnormality, and there are two distinct ways in which the abnormality can arise. The most common method occurs when an extra chromosome is added in the 21 position (hence the name Trisomy 21). Under these conditions, the total chromosome count will be 47 chromosomes, instead of the usual 46. This aberration occurs when chromosome pairs fail to separate during the production of the egg or sperm, a condition known as "nondisjunction." The risk that this chromosomal abnormality will occur is greater with advancing maternal age. Trisomy 21 accounts for most of the babies with Down syndrome. But in about 5% of cases, the extra chromosome is added on to another chromosome. This method is known as "translocation." Under these circumstances, the total chromosome count in the affected baby will be the normal 46, but there will be one "compound" chromosome in this number. Either parent can be the carrier of a "balanced translocation." (A carrier of a "balanced translocation" is clinically normal.) The incidence of this type of Down syndrome is not correlated with maternal age. The compound chromosome will exert the same clinical effects as in the baby with 47 chromosomes.

The risk of giving birth to a baby with Down syndrome, due to nondisjunction, rises with maternal age. When a woman is 30 years old, the risk is estimated to be 1 in 800, while at the age of 44 years, this risk can be as high as 1 in 50.

With translocation, the risk of further babies with Down syndrome is 10% when the translocation is carried by the mother and 2.5% when carried by the father.

There are other, very rare, forms of chromosomal disorders that can produce Down syndrome. These, of course, must be taken into account when genetic counseling is given to couples who already have a child with Down syndrome.

Prenatal diagnosis is available at around the 16th week of pregnancy by amniocentesis. Chorionic villus sampling, at 10 to 12 weeks of pregnancy, is another possible means of prenatal diagnosis. A test measuring alpha-fetoprotein levels in the mother's blood around the 16th week of pregnancy can also help the obstetrician to estimate the mother's risk for having a baby with Down syndrome. Trials are under way, at specialized centers, to perfect an ultrasound technique that can detect specific abnormalities early in pregnancy. This test involves visualizing excessive shadowing in the region of the baby's neck. Recently, however, this shadowing has been suggested to occur more commonly only if there is an added associated heart defect.

CHARACTERISTICS

Diagnosis of Down syndrome can be made at birth by the very specific physical characteristics shown by these babies.

Facial features include an upward slant to the eyes with marked epicanthic folds. A small head, noticeably flatter at the back, in association with a short neck is a typical feature. Ears are small, but the tongue is large and has distinctive deep furrows on the surface.

Eye abnormalities can include cataracts, a lazy eye, and nystagmus, although all these abnormalities are not always present in every child with Down syndrome. The majority of children with Down syndrome have white flecks on the iris known as **Brushfield's spots.** These spots cause no problems with vision, but they are a helpful diagnostic feature.

Limbs are relatively short, making final height on the low side of average. Bodily proportions are normal (unlike in achondroplasia).

Fingers are short and stubby, and many babies have a characteristically in-turning little finger. There is usually a single palmar crease. This feature is common in children with some degree of mental retardation, although single palmar creases on the hands can also be found on many people with normal intellectual abilities.

Feet have a specific characteristic: the great toe is widely separated from the other toes. This feature is most obvious when looking at the soles of the feet.

Muscle tone is always poor, so that babies with Down syndrome are usually "floppy" babies. Subsequent physical development is slower than normal, and walking occurs relatively late.

These are the specific characteristics by which a baby with Down syndrome can be recognized at birth. Confirmation will need to be done by chromosomal analysis.

As development proceeds, it becomes obvious that **developmental delay** is present. Intellectual development is often slow in the first few months or years of life, but can be within the range of normal. As the child matures, he/she is seen to be falling further and further behind his/her peers. Schooling can often initially take place in mainstream schools, but by the time secondary-school age is reached, special facilities will be needed if the child is to fulfill his/her full potential.

Personality: children with Down syndrome are affectionate, happy young people who are a delight to have around. They have an inherent sense of fun, which can add much to family life.

Other features are frequently associated with Down syndrome:

- **Congenital heart disease** affects around 40% of babies with Down syndrome. The most common anomalies are atrial septal defects, ventricular septal defects, and/or patent ductus arteriosus. The first noticeable sign of a cardiac problem is sometimes a failure to thrive adequately. Under these conditions, an echocardiogram may show a hitherto unsuspected heart defect.
- **Upper respiratory tract infections** are common throughout infancy and childhood. This problem is in part due to the smallness of the air passages, as well as an impaired immune system. Similarly, ear infections are common and can lead to a conductive deafness.
- **Thyroid disease,** both hypo- and hyperthyroidism, occurs in about 20% of children with Down syndrome. Hypothyroidism is the most common disease.
- **Acute lymphatic leukemia** affects children with Down syndrome more often than other children and is responsible for around 5% of deaths in early childhood.

MANAGEMENT IMPLICATIONS

Mental handicap: This consistent feature of children with Down syndrome needs careful assessment and management. The infant and young child will be maturing along the same lines as his/her peers, although at a progressively slower rate. Therefore, it is important that suitable playthings for the developmental stage reached, and not the chronological age, should be provided.

Physical therapy help is important in the early life of the child with Down syndrome. Help can be given to encourage movement and to advise parents on the management of their hypotonic baby. The activities suggested will also help to control the recurrent respiratory tract infections to which babies with Down syndrome are particularly susceptible.

Attendance at a play group and nursery school can follow the usual pattern, and many children with Down syndrome manage very adequately in the lower classes of the mainstream school. By the age of about seven or eight years, however, it becomes obvious that the child is finding the work difficult. His/her small stature, poor coordination, and relatively weak muscles all make it difficult for the child to participate with his/her peers. At this time, comprehensive assessment to determine the way forward is greatly important. Some type of special schooling, or extra resources, will usually be needed. The type of education will depend very much on available local options.

Children with Down syndrome should ideally live as part of a normal family. Their affectionate, happy personality flowers within the love and security of the family unit.

Eye abnormalities: lazy eyes need to be assessed and correction undertaken, by orthoptic or surgical means, if amblyopia is to be avoided. Avoiding this condition is important, as children with Down syndrome need all possible sensory input to maximize their abilities.

Respiratory tract infections, which are frequently associated with middle ear infection, will need adequate and sustained treatment. Bronchitis, following on from upper respiratory tract infections, is common in children with Down syndrome, and it will demand adequate treatment.

Deafness, as a result of frequent middle ear disease, needs assessment and treatment. Distraction tests are usually successful in assessing hearing. Myringotomy, to remove sticky secretions from the middle ear, may be all that is necessary in the early stages, although many children with Down syndrome will need hearing aids later in life.

Thyroid disease must always be remembered when caring for a child with Down syndrome. Any excessive slowing of activity with weight gain, specific hair loss, and a hoarse voice should alert care givers to the possibility of hypothyroidism. Treatment with thyroxine will remedy this condition. Routine assessment of thyroid function throughout life is necessary to maintain the correct level of this hormone.

Congenital heart disease can be noted during routine medical checks. If a defect has been found, regular follow-up, and appropriate treatment if necessary, should be done.

Weight control is also important for the child with Down syndrome. Excess weight is often gained due to the relative immobility of these children. Dietary advice is valuable.

THE FUTURE

If the first year of life is survived, children with Down syndrome have an average life expectancy of around 40 to 50 years, although ages of over 60 have been attained. Mortality during the first year of life is usually due to congenital heart disease and/or respiratory tract infections. Malignancies, particularly leukemia, account for deaths later in childhood.

Work in a sheltered environment, or attendance at a special center where suitable occupations are available, can be undertaken by adults with Down syndrome. Lives can be happy and fulfilled within such a caring environment.

It is believed that all men with Down syndrome are infertile, and women have a low fertility.

In later life, features of Alzheimer's disease can unhappily make their appearance, adding to the difficulties of caring for these older people with Down syndrome.

SELF-HELP GROUPS

National Down Syndrome Society
666 Broadway
New York, NY 10012-2317
800-221-4602 or 212-460-9330
http://www.ndss.org
email: info@ndss.org

National Down Syndrome Congress
7000 Peachtree-Dunwood Road, N.E.
Lake Ridge 4000 Office Park
Building 5, Suite 100
Atlanta, GA 30328
770-604-9500 or 800-232-6372
http://members.carol.net/~ndsc
email: ndsccenter@aol.com

Duchenne Muscular Dystrophy

ALTERNATIVE NAMES

Childhood pseudohypertrophic muscular dystrophy; progressive muscular dystrophy.

INCIDENCE

The disease affects males only. In the USA, Australia, and Japan the average incidence of Duchenne muscular dystrophy is thought to be 1 in every 3,300 live-born boys.

There are a number of other neuromuscular disorders that have similar characteristics, but Duchenne muscular dystrophy is by far the most common type to be found in childhood.

HISTORY

The typical signs and symptoms of Duchenne muscular dystrophy were described as long ago as 1861. In 1943, the X-linked pattern of inheritance was determined; in 1983, the exact site of the gene on the X chromosome was located.

CAUSATION

Duchenne muscular dystrophy is inherited, usually as an X-linked recessive condition; therefore, only boys are affected, with about two-thirds of their mothers being carriers. New mutations can also give rise to the condition. The basic fault is the defect of a specific protein found in muscle fibers, known as "dystrophin." The absence of this protein in specific parts of the muscle probably allows leakage of specific enzymes, such as creatine kinase, into the bloodstream. The presence of high levels of creatine kinase in a blood sample of an affected child is confirmation of Duchenne muscular dystrophy.

Prenatal diagnosis begins by determining the sex of the baby. If the baby is a boy, then prenatal DNA studies can be done at around 10 weeks of pregnancy.

Genetic counseling is important for families with a boy affected by Duchenne muscular dystrophy.

CHARACTERISTICS

Boys with Duchenne muscular dystrophy have no signs of the disease at birth, and they develop and grow normally until they are around 18 months old. Between that age and three years, the characteristic clinical features of the condition make their appearance.

Walking: there may be some delay in the onset of this skill—the boy may be 18 months old or older before he walks. (Of course, the normal age at which children learn to walk varies considerably, ranging from nine months to two years old. Nevertheless, any boy who is not showing definite signs of being able to walk at 18 months should be carefully watched for further signs of Duchenne muscular dystrophy.)

By three years of age, the diagnosis is usually obvious. The boy will have a waddling gait with a marked **lumbar lordosis** and will still fall frequently. He will have great difficulty in running, if he can run at all, and he will also find climbing stairs a problem. The classical sign of Duchenne muscular dystrophy occurs as the affected boy tries to get up onto his feet after a fall. He will push his legs out behind him, while placing his hands on the floor in front. He will then "walk" his hands up to his legs to push himself into the upright position. This process is known as the "Gower maneuver." The difficulties in walking and associated activities are due to weakness of the pelvic and leg muscles. The muscles of the calves of the legs of boys with Duchenne muscular dystrophy are often enlarged, giving the false appearance of power. This enlargement is due to an infiltration of the muscle by fibrous and fatty tissue. (This condition is the reason behind the alternative name of pseudohypertrophic muscular dystrophy.) The tendons at the heel (i.e., the Achilles' tendon) are tight in boys with muscular dystrophy, and this condition adds to the walking difficulties.

Other **muscles** of the body become progressively involved in the disease process. Muscles of the shoulders, arms, and chest become weakened, and movements of all kinds become more and more difficult.

Chest deformities and **scoliosis** can occur, and **breathing** eventually becomes affected due to the weakness of the intercostal muscles that are closely involved in the normal breathing process. Due to this involvement of the respiratory muscles, bronchitis and pneumonia are more likely to affect children with Duchenne muscular dystrophy than other children.

The **heart muscle** is not exempt from the generalized musculature problems, and congestive heart failure can occur.

Specific learning difficulties, dyslexia in particular, can occur in a minority of boys with Duchenne muscular dystrophy. It is thought that about one-third of boys with the condition may have this added problem.

INVESTIGATIONS

Specific investigations are available to confirm the clinical diagnosis of Duchenne muscular dystrophy:

- **Creatine kinase** levels in the blood are very high, often up to 10 times the normal level for this enzyme. These high levels are always present in the very earliest stages of the disease. Over the succeeding years, the level falls but never reaches normal values.
- **EKG** abnormalities are seen in the tracing in 70 to 90% of boys with Duchenne muscular dystrophy.
- **Electromyelogram** and **muscle biopsy** of affected muscles are always found to be abnormal.

Regrettably, Duchenne muscular dystrophy is a progressive disease, and boys with the disease become wheelchair-bound by the time they reach 10 to 12 years of age. Death from respiratory infection or cardiac failure is the usual tragic outcome by the early twenties or before.

MANAGEMENT IMPLICATIONS

There is at present no cure for Duchenne muscular dystrophy, but much can be done to improve the quality of life for the boy with the disease.

Moderate **exercise** within the limits of possible movement is important in the early years of the disease. Exercise that is too strenuous should be avoided, however, as this exertion will only accelerate the breakdown of muscle tissue. Immobilization of any kind will lead to the risk of joint contractures and also may encourage obesity, which in turn will add to respiratory problems. Physical therapy is of immense value and should be given top priority in the early stages of the condition. Passive stretching of hip, knee, and ankle joints should be done, and parents should be taught how to continue these exercises on a regular basis. Similarly, good breathing habits should be taught, and boys (and their parents!) encouraged to practice these habits on a regular, daily basis.

Later, as the disease inexorably progresses, a suitable **wheelchair** will be necessary. Electrically propelled chairs will make the child more self-sufficient once he is able to manage this piece of equipment. Attention must be paid to the correct size of the wheelchair. The seating part of the chair is of particular importance in the prevention of scoliosis and all its possible attendant chest problems.

Skin care is especially important because the loss of muscle bulk and accompanying weight loss can make the skin very fragile.

Home modifications for sleeping and toileting purposes may need to be considered as the child matures.

Schooling in special, wheelchair-accessible facilities must be organized. The boy with Duchenne muscular dystrophy will need to be encouraged to take interest in nonphysical activities. The help of an occupational therapist is also of value for this purpose.

Lung infections and possible **heart failure** must receive urgent and ongoing medical attention.

Constipation can be a minor, but irritating, problem of life in a wheelchair. Diet, with perhaps a suitable occasional medication for this purpose, should be successful in eliminating this uncomfortable problem.

Support from a specialist social worker is valuable. Financial assistance can be sorted out, and short-term residential care to allow other members of the family an active vacation may possibly be arranged.

Emotional support for the family from all involved, in whatever capacity, is a very real necessity. The progressive nature of the disease, with the very poor life expectancy, can make coming to terms with the facts extremely difficult. Both parents and the boy will all need continuing, sensitive support, especially if another boy in the family has already died from the condition, or there is a family member who is in a later stage of the disease.

THE FUTURE

Life in a wheelchair from around 10 to 12 years old, and an early death from cardiac or respiratory failure, is the depressing outlook for boys with Duchenne muscular dystrophy. However, a positive approach with adequate support can vastly improve the quality of life for the whole family.

SELF-HELP GROUP

Muscular Dystrophy Association—USA
National Headquarters
3300 E. Sunrise Drive
Tucson, AZ 85718
800-572-1717
http://www.mdausa.org

Edwards Syndrome

ALTERNATIVE NAME

Trisomy 18.

INCIDENCE

In the USA and UK, the incidence of Edwards syndrome is reported to be 1 in every 6,600 live births. Edwards syndrome is a chromosomal abnormality, which can be divided into three groups according to the severity of the condition.

- The most severe form, where the majority of cells in the body show the abnormality. The baby is severely handicapped and has only a very short life expectancy.
- The "mosaic" form, in which some cells in the body have a normal chromosome complement while others have the typical chromosomal pattern of the severe form of Edwards syndrome. These babies are less severely affected and have a longer life expectancy.
- A milder, or partial, form of the condition, depending on the part of the chromosome affected. These babies can show few signs of abnormality and will only have minimal handicap.

Girls are marginally more often affected than boys by Edwards syndrome.

CAUSATION

Babies born with Edwards syndrome have 47 chromosomes instead of the usual complement of 46. The extra chromosome is in the 18 position (cf. Down syndrome). Older mothers seem to be at higher risk than younger mothers of having babies born with Edwards syndrome.

The actual mode of inheritance is not entirely clear, but it is thought that the mosaic form may be directly inherited—the other types occurring sporadically.

Chorionic villus sampling can diagnose the syndrome at 9 to 12 weeks of pregnancy, while amniocentesis at 16 weeks shows the unusual chromosome count in the aspirated amniotic fluid. During the pregnancy of a baby with Edwards syndrome, there is frequently an excess of amniotic fluid. The fetus tends to move less than does a normal fetus during the latter months of pregnancy. Also, such pregnancies often tend to last longer than the usual 40 weeks. It is important that chromosomal analysis is done on the cells of an affected fetus to be certain of the diagnosis. The serious implications of the finding of an extra chromosome 18 can then be faced and appropriate care and support of the family given.

CHARACTERISTICS

These can be multiple, and many of the manifestations can be found in other syndromes. It is therefore important that all the features are considered together before a definite diagnosis is made, supported eventually by chromosomal analysis.

All babies with the severe form of trisomy 18 are **developmentally delayed** with severe **mental handicap**. Other babies with the mosaic or partial forms may have varying degrees of mental handicap or have normal intellectual abilities.

Many of the babies are **hypotonic** at birth, and this condition can cause **feeding difficulties** because of the baby's inability to suck adequately. As a result of these difficulties, weight gain and growth in general are slow.

After the neonatal period has passed, babies with Edwards syndrome become **hypertonic.**

As many as 95% of severely affected babies have a **congenital heart defect:** ventricular septal defects and patent ductus arteriosus are the two most commonly seen abnormalities.

Hands and **feet** both show very specific abnormalities. The baby with Edwards syndrome usually holds his fists tightly clenched with the fourth and fifth fingers overlapping the other fingers. There is also often a single palmar crease, and the markings on the finger tips are unusual. Feet are convex on the soles and are termed "rockerbottom" feet. Heels are also particularly prominent, adding to the unusual shape of the feet.

Renal abnormalities are common in babies with Edwards syndrome. Horseshoe kidneys are found in more than 50% of babies. Renal problems may not become apparent within the first few weeks of life or may be so severe as to cause early renal failure.

Facial features include low-set and unusually shaped ears, a short neck, and a small jaw. The diameter between the parietal bones of the skull is small; this measurement can be a diagnostic feature on ultrasound in the prenatal period.

MANAGEMENT IMPLICATIONS

It is vital that the correct diagnosis is made by chromosomal analysis so that parents can be told of the problems that may be encountered as their baby grows. Support and sensitive counseling will be necessary for those parents who have a severely affected baby who is not expected to live more than a few months.

Feeding difficulties will need to be addressed in the early days, and nasogastric feeding may initially be necessary, due to the poor suck and excessive tiring of the hypotonic baby. Feeding with expressed breast milk is advised.

Respiratory difficulties frequently occur and will need specialized treatment in the early days of life.

Congenital heart disease, so commonly found, will need accurate diagnosis and assessment. Incipient cardiac failure must be treated and future surgery contemplated, depending, of course, on the general condition of the baby.

Mental handicap will need to be fully assessed at a later date, and the less seriously affected child should undergo repeated checks of developmental milestones.

THE FUTURE

For babies with the severe form of Edwards syndrome, death usually occurs within the first few weeks or months of life. With the partial form, however, the outlook is less grim. Depending on the severity of the condition, the child may live into the teenage years, or even longer. Handicap will again depend on the severity of the condition.

Following the birth of a baby with Edwards syndrome, genetic counseling for the parents is indicated before a further pregnancy ensues.

SELF-HELP GROUP

SOFT USA
Barb Vanherreweghe
2982 South Union Street
Rochester, NY 14624
716-594-4621 or 800-716-7638
http://www.trisomy.org
email: barb@trisomy.org

Ehlers–Danlos Syndrome

ALTERNATIVE NAME

Joint laxity.

INCIDENCE

Ehlers–Danlos syndrome is very rare. In the UK, incidence is in the region of 1 in every 50,000 live births. The number of cases in other parts of the world has not been accurately assessed.

There are a number of subtypes of Ehlers–Danlos syndrome: nine have been described to date. As research into the condition proceeds, it is possible that a number of further variants will be found. All types have in common some disorder of the connective tissues of the body. Such disorders include problems with skin and joints, but in some types of the syndrome, blood vessels and internal organs can also be affected.

Boys and girls are affected equally by most variants. Only boys are affected by Ehlers–Danlos type 5, due to the mode of inheritance.

HISTORY

International research is being carried out into this syndrome. Much initial work was done in the 1970s and 1980s.

CAUSATION

Ehlers–Danlos syndrome is a genetic condition; most types are inherited as an autosomal dominant. Ehlers–Danlos 5, however, is an X-linked recessive condition.

Routine prenatal diagnosis is not currently available, although gene marker tests are available for some types. Ehlers–Danlos syndrome is not immediately apparent at birth, but it does become noticeable in early childhood.

It is probable that a specific enzyme defect is the basic cause of this syndrome.

CHARACTERISTICS

All types of Ehlers–Danlos syndrome have the following two characteristics.

Joint hypermobility: many of the joints of the body can be put through an extraordinarily wide range of movements. For example, thumbs can easily be pulled back onto the forearm. This hypermobility is primarily due to the laxity of the ligaments surrounding the joints. As a result of this extreme looseness, joints are easily dislocated on minimal injury. In some types of Ehlers–Danlos syndrome, bones become deformed due to the lack of support around the joints by capsules and ligaments. The most obvious example of this type of deformity is probably the extreme flat feet (pes planus) seen in some children and adults with this condition. Severe scoliosis can be a worrying feature of the syndrome, again due to the lack of support around the vertebral joints by ligaments.

The **skin** can be pulled away easily from the underlying tissues and is especially fragile, making injury common with minimal trauma. Bruising occurs frequently, due both to skin fragility and to abnormalities in the walls of the underlying blood vessels. Damage to skin is particularly likely to occur over bony prominences, such as elbows and knees, and also in places where skin is stretched tightly over underlying bones, such as the shins and the forehead. Wounds can take longer than usual to heal, due to general tissue fragility. Scars are paper-thin, making the person with Ehlers–Danlos syndrome prone to recurrent injury.

Other problems encountered in different subtypes of Ehlers–Danlos syndrome include the following.

- **Arteries:** in one type of this syndrome, these important blood vessels are especially affected. The walls are thin and easily ruptured. This situation is a potentially dangerous and can lead to fatalities.
- **Teeth** and the surrounding gums are especially affected in another type of this syndrome. Teeth become loose at an early age due to repeated gum infections, forcing the extraction of teeth.
- **Eyes** can be affected by the generalized disorder of connective tissue. Detachment of the retina, which can lead to rapid loss of vision if it is not treated urgently, is common.

All of these effects are not necessarily to be found in any one child suffering from Ehlers–Danlos syndrome. The subtype present determines which connective tissues are predominantly affected.

MANAGEMENT IMPLICATIONS

Joint and skeletal effects: due to the ease with which joints can dislocate, contact sports and physical activities that put excessive strain on joints should be avoided. Rapid reduction of dislocated joints, when and if dislocation occurs, is important. Scoliosis, if present, will benefit from orthopedic advice, as will flat feet. Physical therapy to strengthen muscles surrounding joints is important.

Skin will need similar careful treatment. Any activity in which skin lacerations or bruising have a high probability of occurring should be avoided as far as is possible. Such activities are, of course, an inevitable part of the rough and tumble of childhood, but preventative measures, such as protective padding or clothing over elbows and knees and other bony prominences, can help the child to avoid at least some of injuries. Sympathetic handling is often needed to persuade the child with Ehlers–Danlos syndrome to wear such protective clothing. If injury to the skin does occur, closure of the wound with tape is the preferred method of treatment. Routine stitching can give rise to further problems with healing. If surgery for any reason has to be undertaken, particular care will be needed to be sure that adequate healing takes place.

Teeth: meticulous and ongoing dental care is vital for children and adults with Ehlers–Danlos syndrome. The probable early loss of teeth associated with some types of the syndrome makes good fitting and maintenance of dentures a priority.

Eyes: if retinal detachment occurs, it must be corrected.

THE FUTURE

Children with Ehlers–Danlos syndrome will need to be protected, as far as possible without compromising their spontaneous energies, from injury. Affected children will need the sympathetic cooperation of their playmates as well as knowledge and understanding of their condition from their teachers. Career advice will need to be geared toward more sedentary occupations.

Pregnancy in women with the syndrome can often result in premature birth, due to early rupture of the membranes, which are involved in the general connective tissue abnormality.

Life expectancy is normal for persons with Ehlers–Danlos syndrome, with the exception of those individuals who have the type in which there is particular fragility of the large blood vessels. In such cases, rupture can lead to a fatal outcome.

SELF-HELP GROUP

Ehlers–Danlos National Foundation
6399 Wilshire Boulevard, Suite 510
Los Angeles, CA 90048
323-651-3038
http://www.ednf.org

Ellis–Van Creveld Syndrome

ALTERNATIVE NAME

Chondroectodermal dysplasia.

INCIDENCE

Ellis–van Creveld syndrome is a rare disorder, which has been reported in many parts of the world. (There is an Amish group of people in Pennsylvania for whom the syndrome is not as rare; the higher rate of incidence in this exceptional case is probably explained by the high rate of intermarriage in this community.) Both sexes are equally affected.

Ultrasound after the 16th week of pregnancy can show the extra fingers on the hands that are a feature of the condition.

HISTORY

This condition was described by Ellis and van Creveld in 1940.

CAUSATION

This syndrome is inherited as an autosomal recessive condition.

CHARACTERISTICS

Short stature is one of the main features of Ellis–van Creveld syndrome. Adult height ranges between 3 feet (90 centimeters) and 5 feet (150 centimeters).

The trunk is of normal proportions. The lack of height is caused by shortening of the arms below the elbows and the legs below the knees. These features are noticeable at birth. These measurements lead to an unbalanced appearance as the child matures (cf. achondroplasia and hypochondroplasia).

As the child starts to walk, **knock-knees** will become very apparent. This condition, together with the short legs, makes for an unusual gait.

Extra fingers are a feature of the condition. The extra fingers are usually well-developed. This feature is somewhat unusual: when extra digits are found in persons unaffected by this syndrome, they are frequently little more than tags of skin.

In a small percentage of babies—about 10%—extra **toes** are also present.

Fingernails and **toenails** are small and underdeveloped at birth and remain so throughout life.

Teeth, which erupt early, are of an unusual rounded barrel shape and are widely spaced. (Some babies are born with teeth already erupted. This condition can sometimes lead to difficulties with breast feeding).

More than half the babies born with this syndrome have a congenital **heart defect.** This problem most frequently takes the form of an atrial septal defect—that is, an opening between the two upper chambers of the heart. The defect can lead to heart failure within the first few months of life, which can be fatal. About one-third of babies born with Ellis–van Creveld syndrome die of heart failure within the first few months of life.

MANAGEMENT IMPLICATIONS

Short stature, particularly if the final height is no more than 3 feet, can cause problems, both at school and in later life. Chairs and tables at school will need to be adjusted to suit the child's lack of height.

Sensitive handling is necessary when sports and other physical activities are undertaken. Very short children can become extremely frustrated by their inability to keep up with all the activities that their peers seem to so enjoy. Both parents and teachers should to try to find suitable and enjoyable hobbies for the child with Ellis–van Creveld syndrome.

Later in life, many few commonplace objects will cause problems for the adult of short stature.

Extra **fingers**—and toes, if present,—will need to be surgically removed at some time during the early years, certainly before school days arrive.

Surgery to repair the congenital **heart defect** will be necessary as soon as the baby is strong enough to withstand this procedure.

If **knock-knees** are very marked and make walking difficult, orthopedic advice will be necessary and operative procedures may possibly be required. Following such an operation, physical therapy to strengthen weak muscles and to encourage good posture and walking patterns will be valuable.

Genetic counseling is advisable before parents with one affected child pursue another pregnancy.

THE FUTURE

If there are no cardiac lesions or if these have been dealt with successfully, life expectancy is good. Careers where short stature is not a problem need to be investigated as adulthood approaches. Genetic advice is necessary before pregnancy.

SELF-HELP GROUP

Human Growth Foundation
997 Glen Cove Avenue
Glen Head, NY 11545
800-451-6434
http://www.hgfound.org
email: hgfl@hgfound.org

Epidermolysis Bullosa

ALTERNATIVE NAMES

There are a number of subtypes of this condition, such as epidermolysis bullosa Mendes da Costa and epidermolysis bullosa Koebner type; all subtypes have the prefix "epidermolysis bullosa" or EBS.

INCIDENCE

The true incidence of epidermolysis bullosa is not entirely clear. In the USA, a specific number of large families have been documented in which many family members have the condition. From these studies, it is estimated that there are at least 50,000 Americans (mainly children) suffering from epidermolysis bullosa.

CAUSATION

Most types of EBS are inherited as an autosomal dominant. However, EBS lethal type is inherited in an autosomal recessive manner, and EBS Mendes da Costa is an X-linked recessive condition. The latter subtype only affects boys. In the other types, boys and girls can be equally affected.

At present, there is no prenatal diagnosis available apart from sampling fetal skin at around 18 weeks of pregnancy. Genetic counseling is advisable if there is a family history of the condition.

CHARACTERISTICS

This condition only affects the **skin** and can clinically be divided into a "simple" type and a "dystrophic" type, depending on which layer of the skin is involved. Both types result in blistering from minimal injury.

In the **simple** type, there is a wide variation in the degree of injury that produces blistering. Some babies may arrive in the world with a blistered skin caused by the trauma of delivery. In other babies, it is not until the crawling stage that any problems are encountered. In the latter circumstance, the movements of clothing, particularly on knees and elbows, when crawling is sufficient to cause blistering. Scarring does not occur in this type.

In the **dystrophic** type, the degree of trauma again varies greatly from individual to individual. In this type of EBS, scarring is the usual outcome after healing. The scarring can be severe, giving rise to contractures and the possible loss of finger- and toenails.

Depending on the subtype, blistering may occur anywhere on the body or be confined to the extremities.

The **mucous membrane** in the mouth may be involved in the young baby, but, fortunately, this condition does usually improve in later childhood. Soft, mashed foods should be given for as long as the condition in the mouth is severe.

Problems can arise when blisters become infected; such infections can occur all too readily during the active, "into everything" toddler years.

Other abnormalities can include **erosions and narrowing of the esophagus,** which can give rise to difficulties with swallowing.

Contractures in the joints can occur in some children with epidermolysis bullosa. This condition can cause a degree of disability later in life.

MANAGEMENT IMPLICATIONS

The mainstay of coping with a child with EBS is the avoidance of injury as far as possible. The unavoidable bumps and falls of childhood cause greater problems than normal. The resultant blistering must be treated with great care to avoid infection. Children's skin differs from that of adults because children are less resistant to certain bacteria, making infection is a greater hazard. With increasing maturity, blistering tends to improve and susceptibility to infection diminishes.

School teachers should be alerted to the dangers to which their pupils with EBS are exposed following even minor injury. Professional advice is a wise move if injury does occur at school. Teachers should remember that the usual adhesive bandage designed for minor wounds should never be used on a child with EBS because the removal of the protective dressing will painfully damage the abnormal skin.

An **adequate intake of food** must be maintained for the child with severe EBS. It is all too easy for nutritional deficiencies to arise due to eating problems in the early years. Children do not take readily to eating an adequate diet when their mouths are sore and eating is painful.

Sports with much physical contact are unsuitable for children with EBS. Other activities, such as swimming, dancing, and routine exercises are better for, and enjoyed by, these children.

Many everyday facets of life can be affected by EBS: for example, ironing can present a problem to the child with the disease, as the act of exerting pressure on an iron is sufficient in many cases to cause blistering with all its potential problems. Antibiotic creams will help reduce the possible dangers of infection in a blistered lesion to a minimum.

Brushing teeth can cause blistering and soreness of the gums. A soft toothbrush should be used. Good dental care is vital, and teeth should be preserved in the mouth at all costs because a person with EBS cannot wear dentures.

Itching can sometimes be a feature of EBS, especially if the child becomes too hot. It is important to avoid overheating; an antihistamine may reduce the irritation.

THE FUTURE

EBS does tend to improve with maturity. Also, as they grow older, individuals with EBS learn how to avoid the injuries that are likely to cause blistering.

Career prospects will be limited, depending on the severity of the disease. For example, repetitive work requiring the continual handling of objects will need to be avoided. Sheltered workshops or suitable work from home should be investigated.

Life expectancy is not diminished by EBS (except for the lethal form, in which death occurs in infancy).

SELF-HELP GROUP

DebRA of America, Inc.
40 Rector Street, Suite 1403
New York, NY 10006
212-513-4090
http://www.debra.org
email: staff@debra.org

Fabry Disease

Fabry–Anderson disease; angiokeratoma; alphagalactosidase A deficiency.

INCIDENCE

Due to the complicated inheritance pattern, the exact incidence of Fabry disease is unknown, but it is thought to be about 1 in every 40,000 live births. All races have reported the condition among their populations, with the exception of American Indians. The disease usually affects only boys; reports of symptoms in carrier girls are very rare.

CAUSATION

Fabry disease is a metabolic condition in which there is a defective activity of a specific enzyme concerned with the metabolism of certain lipids in the body. As a result of this defect, there is excessive deposition of these specific lipids in the walls of the blood vessels and also in other parts of the body. This excess in turn gives rise to the symptoms seen in this disease.

Fabry disease is inherited as an X-linked recessive condition. There is a wide variety in the severity of the symptoms in each individual. In rare instances, carrier girls can be affected; their symptoms may range from completely absent to severe.

The condition can be diagnosed prenatally by chorionic villus sampling or by amniocentesis.

CHARACTERISTICS

The first signs of Fabry disease are usually seen in childhood. The child will complain of **pain,** felt first in fingers and toes and then extending up the arms and legs, and, in some cases, across the abdomen and in the genital region. The pain is described as tingling or burning in character and can be very severe. The length of time during which these very unpleasant symptoms last varies from minutes to weeks. There may be a low-grade fever associated with each episode of pain. These painful events are often triggered by excessive tiredness, by an intercurrent infection, or even by a rapid change in environmental temperature, such as coming into a hot room after being outdoors in the cold. Children with these symptoms often will ask to go outside again. These periodic attacks of pain tend to become less frequent during adolescence and adult life. Many people with Fabry disease will complain of permanent discomfort in hands and feet. This condition is often said to be worse in the late afternoon and evening than in other parts of the day.

Skin: at around the same time as these unpleasant sensations occur, clusters of dark red spots known as angiokeratomas, make their appearance. They can occur anywhere on the body, but they are most typically seen in the greatest number on the lower part of the trunk and the upper part of the legs.

Eyes: in later childhood, opaque areas, arising in whorls, can be seen on the cornea upon examination under a slitlamp. Depending on their severity, these opaque areas can cause a degree of blurred vision. In addition to these opacities, dilated and tortuous blood vessels course over the conjunctiva. In an ophthalmoscopic examination, similarly damaged blood vessels can be seen in the retina.

Renal complications due to the involvement of the blood vessels of the kidney can occur in late childhood and early adult life. There is gradual deterioration of kidney function, and renal failure can occur at any time from the 10th birthday onward.

Heart: the coronary blood vessels are involved in the generalized abnormality caused by the enzyme defect, and persons with the syndrome may face coronary heart disease. Valvular heart disease, most frequently a prolapse of the mitral valve, is also associated frequently with Fabry disease.

Similarly, **strokes** can occur from damaged cerebral blood vessels.

Other more unusual symptoms can include:

- nausea, vomiting, diarrhea, and abdominal pain, due to depositions of abnormal lipids in the abdominal tissues;
- Perthes disease, due to avascular necrosis of the head of the femur;
- delay in normal growth and in puberty in severely affected boys;
- excessive fatigue and weakness throughout childhood in those severely affected; and
- in severely affected children, chronic breathing difficulties caused by the obstructive accumulation of specific substances in the lining of the airways.

The symptoms and signs of Fabry disease can be wide-ranging and severe, leading to a good deal of difficulty in diagnosis. Finding very high levels of the specific substances that are being incompletely metabolized can lead to a firm diagnosis.

MANAGEMENT IMPLICATIONS

The **painful episodes** in limbs and other parts of the body can be relieved by giving certain specific drugs, such as carbamazepine. Ensuring that children do not become too hot or overtired and avoiding, as far as possible, sudden changes in environmental temperature will also help reduce the number of incidents of pain.

Children and parents can be reassured that as they get older these episodes will become less frequent.

The **renal and heart complications** that can occur in later childhood need to be treated appropriately. Renal dialysis and kidney transplantation may be necessary in later life.

THE FUTURE

Until kidney transplantation became available, renal failure often led to death when the affected person was in his forties. Transplants can now prolong life expectancy, unless the heart is severely affected, or a stroke is suffered.

Within the limits of disability, most careers can be followed, except those in which extreme ranges of temperature are found.

Enzyme replacement therapy is being researched, and in the future, it will perhaps, lead to a cure for Fabry disease.

SELF-HELP GROUP

Fabry Support and Information Group
P.O. Box 569
Concordia, MO 64020-0569
660-463-1382

Fetal Alcohol Syndrome

INCIDENCE

The incidence of this syndrome varies from place to place, depending on the drinking habits of the local population. If the drinking habits of the mother during pregnancy are very heavy, nutrition will also have an effect on the development of the baby.

Genetic susceptibility is also thought to have an effect on the incidence of this syndrome.

HISTORY

The specific characteristics shown by babies born to mothers who drink heavily during pregnancy have only been described in detail fairly recently. The amount of alcohol needed to be consumed before demonstrable effects are seen in the baby is not clearly determined. The result will also depend on both mother's and baby's susceptibility to the effects of alcohol.

CAUSATION

Alcohol, and its derivatives, can cross the placenta and exert damaging effects on the developing fetus. The fetus, which does not have available the enzymes necessary to "detoxify" these substances readily, will be susceptible to their adverse effects long after the alcohol has been eliminated from the mother's system. In addition to this direct effect, there can be other indirect problems. Malnutrition, dehydration, and a poorly functioning placenta—all due to excess alcohol intake—can add to the adverse effects of alcohol.

Developmental problems arise early in pregnancy (often before the mother herself is even aware that she is pregnant), when maximum formation of vital organs occurs. The severity of the problem will depend on both the timing of alcohol consumption during the pregnancy and the amount of alcohol consumed. Therefore, it is important that drinking habits are controlled in all women who may expect to become pregnant in the foreseeable future. Defects due to this condition are probably one of the most obviously preventable causes of mental retardation.

CHARACTERISTICS

Small size: babies who are born to mothers who drink heavily are often small for dates (i.e., they weigh less than would be expected for the length of pregnancy). They are frequently born prematurely. These babies grow slowly during the early months, not "catching up" on weight and length as do most premature babies.

Facial features are quite specific for babies born with the fetal alcohol syndrome. The forehead is narrow, often with small eyes and drooping eyelids, which give a sleepy appearance. The top lip is long and smooth, without the "rosebud" appearance common in babies. The lower jaw can be small.

Mental retardation frequently, but not invariably, occurs.

Many babies are **irritable** during the early weeks. They can later become hyperactive and easily distracted. **Speech delay** has also been reported.

The extremity of these effects varies widely, but all children exposed to excess levels of alcohol prenatally will show developmental delay and will probably not reach their full genetic potential.

Hearing may be affected, as there is sometimes a specific malfunction of the Eustachian tube, that tiny tube linking the back of the throat with the middle ear.

Babies with fetal alcohol syndrome have been noted to be very **hairy** at birth; **lazy eyes** are common; and increased susceptibility to **infections** of all kinds has been noted.

MANAGEMENT IMPLICATIONS

Small size: children with the fetal alcohol syndrome will grow along the lower percentiles of the growth charts, and there is little that can be done to accelerate growth. This problem persists throughout childhood.

Mental retardation: close watch must be kept on all aspects of development. The fact that the child lags behind in some aspects of the normal developmental process can be the first clue to diagnosis and to subsequent development. Fuller assessment of areas of detected delay should be undertaken and appropriate help given to ensure that the child's full potential is reached. Speech therapy is frequently needed for speech delay.

Infections of all kinds, but most usually those connected with the respiratory tract, need to be swiftly and adequately treated whenever they occur.

Hearing must be routinely checked, and continued to be monitored on a regular basis, due to the potential Eustachian tube problems. Such check-ups are especially necessary following a cold.

General care and nutrition of babies born to mothers with an alcohol problem must always be at the forefront of the health professionals' minds. The mother may need help both to overcome her drinking problem and to care adequately for her child. Health and social workers should cooperate fully to ensure that the child's safety, health, and development are not adversely affected by a parent's alcohol problem.

THE FUTURE

The child's future is very much dependent upon the care received during infancy and childhood as well as the degree of severity of the alcohol effects.

Also, unless parents can be persuaded to give up their excessive drinking habits, the child, by imitation, can easily grow up to abuse alcohol. Much education needs to be done on the adverse effects of heavy drinking during pregnancy.

SELF-HELP GROUPS

National Organization on Fetal Alcohol Syndrome
418 C Street, N.E.
Washington, DC 20002
202-785-4585
http://www.nofas.org
email: nofas@erols.com

Fetal Alcohol Syndrome Family Resource Institute
P.O. Box 2525
Lynwood, WA 98036
253-531-2878
http://www.accessone.com
email: delindam@accessone.com

Fragile X Syndrome

ALTERNATIVE NAMES

Martin–Bell X-linked mental retardation; fragile X chromosome.

INCIDENCE

It is thought that mental retardation due to fragile X syndrome occurs in approximately 1 in every 2,000 to 3,000 male births. This figure is very high, and this syndrome is therefore thought to be one of the most common causes of mental retardation in boys. Girls are also affected, but to a lesser degree due to the mode of inheritance. Only 30 to 40% of girls carrying this genetic abnormality will have some degree of mental retardation.

HISTORY

In 1943, Martin and Bell first published accounts of a sex-linked form of mental retardation. In the late 1960s, Lubs first described a family with the characteristics now known to be associated with fragile X syndrome. The genetics of this abnormality have subsequently been demonstrated. Boys with mental retardation associated with few other physical features were previously termed as having "pure" mental retardation.

There are a number of other syndromes of a similar type linked in some way to the X chromosome. Clinical features vary in these other syndromes, but mental retardation of some degree is a constant finding.

CAUSATION

The cause of fragile X syndrome is a genetic defect in a particular "fragile" part of the X chromosome (one of the sex chromosomes). The actual genetic transmission is complicated and has not, as yet, been clearly resolved. Many families with a child with fragile X syndrome show a definite X-linked pattern of inheritance (i.e., the condition is passed on from a carrier mother to an affected son). Many sporadic cases are now being recognized, but they may be variations of other X-linked syndromes.

At present, there is no reliable prenatal test, although chorionic villus sampling in the tenth week of pregnancy can detect fragile X syndrome in affected boys.

CHARACTERISTICS

Mental retardation: the degree of this characteristic varies markedly from child to child. Some children are severely retarded, while others have IQs on the borderline of normal. For example, a child may have only mild difficulties with reading or mathematical concepts. On the other hand, some boys can be so severely affected that characteristics such as hyperactivity, repetitive behavior, autistic features, hand-flapping, and speech difficulties occur. Girls with fragile X syndrome (as confirmed by chromosome studies) usually have normal intelligence, although a few may be mildly retarded.

Testes in 90% of boys with fragile X syndrome become larger than normal at puberty. This condition may affect one testicle only. There does not appear to be any loss of normal testicular function, although few affected men have been known to father children.

Facial features: a long, thin face is frequently associated with fragile X syndrome in both boys and girls. Boys tend to have large ears and a prominent forehead.

The following features can also occur, and their presence may aid diagnosis.

Speech is frequently specifically delayed during the early years. This problem can be part of the general developmental delay seen as the child matures.

Fingers that are easily hyperextended, due to the loose connective tissue around the joints, are often a feature of children with fragile X syndrome.

Skin is often fine and thin.

MANAGEMENT IMPLICATIONS

All babies benefit from physical and verbal stimulation during the early growing years. Such stimulation is particularly important for those children with **potential developmental delay.** Care givers should talk to babies from birth onward, even if no obvious response is forthcoming. Similarly, simple games that encourage coordination of hands and limbs will help children develop to their full potential. Help in these areas is of particular importance to children with fragile X syndrome.

Help from clinical psychologists can be of value in the early years if autistic or hyperactive behavior is a problem.

Comprehensive multidisciplinary assessment, on an ongoing basis, is vital to determine those areas of development in which the child is lagging behind. Where problems are detected, appropriate help can then be given in the areas of delay.

Boys will probably need special schooling facilities, although some boys manage quite adequately in mainstream schools if additional help is available. Again, full multidisciplinary assessment is necessary to determine the most appropriate placement.

Genetic counseling for families who have a member with a proven case of fragile X syndrome is important.

THE FUTURE

Career and job prospects will be limited for boys with severe mental retardation. Sheltered employment in a caring community or with full support from a loving home is the best option under these circumstances. For the less severely affected boys, and certainly for girls with this genetic abnormality, a wide variety of work is possible.

Life expectancy for children with fragile X syndrome is not limited.

SELF-HELP GROUP

National Fragile X Foundation
P.O. Box 190488
San Francisco, CA 94119
800-688-8765 or 510-763-6030
http://www.nfxf.org

Friedrich Ataxia

ALTERNATIVE NAMES

Friedrich disease; hereditary spinal ataxia; recessive spinocerebellar degeneration.

INCIDENCE

There are a number of conditions that have ataxia as the prime characteristic. Friedrich ataxia is thought to be the most common of the hereditary ataxias. Approximately 1 baby in 50,000 is likely to be affected. Boys and girls can be affected equally.

HISTORY

The most recent work on the basic cause of Friedrich ataxia has been done by Harding. Suggestions have been made that the disease may be a metabolic one. This supposition differs greatly from Friedrich's original thoughts on the matter, which were that the disease was due to alcoholic excess.

Active research into Friedrich ataxia is currently being undertaken, and much work needs to be done to differentiate this form of ataxia from other conditions with somewhat similar symptoms.

CAUSATION

Friedrich ataxia is inherited as an autosomal recessive characteristic. The gene affected is situated on chromosome 9. The pathology is one of atrophy of specific parts of the spinal cord.

Prenatal diagnosis can be made by chorionic villus sampling at 8 to 12 weeks of pregnancy. Genetic counseling is advisable for families who have a member with Friedrich ataxia.

CHARACTERISTICS

Ataxia is the most obvious characteristic of this condition. At birth and up to around the age of three years, there are no signs at all of any problem. In fact, the age at which the disease first manifests itself is very variable, and, in some children, symptoms only develop at puberty. The unsteadiness develops first in the legs and ascends relentlessly up the body until all four limbs are affected. Accompanying this unsteadiness is weakness and an inability for the child to determine the position of her/his limbs in space, which adds to the ataxic problems. Sensations of touch are also diminished, but both pain and temperature change can be felt normally. Reflexes in the legs are lost early, and the plantar response is extensor. Regrettably, most persons with Friedrich ataxia will be wheelchair-bound by the time they are 25 years old.

Eyes: nystagmus or other disturbances of eye movements are noticeable in about half the children with Friedrich ataxia. Optic atrophy also can occur in a minority of affected persons.

Deafness, although less commonly seen than other abnormalities, can add to the problems of persons with Friedrich ataxia.

Scoliosis and **flat feet** develop within a few years of the disease becoming obvious. These effects arise gradually over the years as the ataxic gait becomes more apparent.

Heart: the heart is always eventually affected in Friedrich ataxia. This vital organ becomes hypertrophied (enlarged), causing it to function less well. Breathlessness and palpitations are the symptoms most usually felt by the young person. EKG changes become obvious and show left ventricular hypertrophy and T-wave inversion as the condition progresses.

Diabetes develops in a significant number (20%) of those persons affected by a later stage of Friedrich ataxia. The development of this metabolic condition is more likely to occur in those children and young adults with visual and hearing problems.

MANAGEMENT IMPLICATIONS

Ataxia: the child with problems of unsteadiness when walking will need to be protected against injury from falls during the early stage of the disease. Progressive weakness of the muscles will make many physical activities difficult or impossible. Depending on the severity and rate of progression of the condition, a wheelchair will probably become an eventual necessity.

Physical therapy, both to reduce as far as possible skeletal deformities and to keep weakened muscles on the move, is valuable. Many sufferers have commented that bed rest seems to make their condition worse. Therefore, confinement to bed during any bout of intercurrent infection should be reduced to a minimum.

Speech therapy can help boys and girls to find the best way to use the muscles of articulation that are affected by the disease.

Vision and **hearing** must be monitored on a continuing basis. For example, any associated refractory defect or conductive deafness due to infection should be treated early and adequately.

Heart: cardiac function needs to be accurately assessed clinically and by EKG, and maybe also by echocardiography. Digoxin and / or betablocker drugs are often helpful in maintaining adequate cardiac function.

Diabetes: the fact that this metabolic condition is strongly associated with Friedrich ataxia must be remembered. Symptoms of thirst, frequent urination, and loss of weight must be urgently investigated, and appropriate treatment must be given if blood sugar levels are found to be high.

Skeletal problems of scoliosis may be so severe as to need surgery. The deformed chest, due to the spinal "twist," can give rise to problems with respiration.

THE FUTURE

Friedrich ataxia unfortunately pursues a relentless course with few, if any, periods of remission. Few individuals with this ataxia remain out of a wheelchair by the time the early twenties are reached. A fatal outcome usually occurs before the fortieth birthday, most frequently from cardiac complications or an intercurrent respiratory infection. These events can vary, however, and life expectancy is enhanced for those people with less severe symptoms (especially for persons with only mild cardiac symptoms and without diabetes). Improvements in treatment of cardiac and diabetic problems have, in recent years, resulted in greater longevity.

Career choices are limited by the degree to which the ataxia affects large muscle groups and the muscles of articulation.

SELF-HELP GROUP

National Ataxia Foundation
2600 Fernbrook Lane, Suite 119
Minneapolis, MN 55447
612-553-0020
http:/ / ataxia.org
email: naf@mr.net

Galactosemia

About 1 baby in every 50,000 born in the UK, the USA, and Germany is affected by this metabolic disease. Ireland and Austria appear to have more babies born with this condition, while Japanese babies are affected very rarely. Both boys and girls can show the characteristics of galactosemia.

CAUSATION

Galactosemia is inherited as an autosomal recessive condition. Chromosome 9 appears to be the chromosome on which the affected gene is located. Chorionic villus sampling at 9 to 12 weeks of pregnancy, followed (if necessary) by amniocentesis a month later, will show deficiency of the enzyme involved in this condition. It is the absence, or deficient production of, this enzyme that gives rise to the characteristic features. Galactose, a substance found in milk and milk products, is the substance that is incompletely broken down. As a result, accumulation of galactose, and other allied substances, is found in various parts of the body in children suffering from this condition.

At birth, blood tests will find that the enzyme involved in the breakdown and proper metabolism of galactose is absent. In the USA, all babies are routinely screened for galactosemia by this method.

CHARACTERISTICS

The baby is entirely well at birth. It is not until milk feedings are given on the second or third day of life that symptoms begin to appear.

The baby will, between four and ten days of age, become **jaundiced,** and she or he will begin to refuse feedings. **Vomiting** will soon become a problem, causing the baby to lose weight and to become lethargic and drowsy.

Overwhelming infection in any part of the body is one of the gravest dangers at this young age. Infections, particularly from E. coli bacteria, are particularly liable to afflict babies with galactosemia. He/she will be gravely ill, and death is an ever-present threat under these conditions. Even if the baby does recover from an infection, mental and physical development can be retarded unless the true cause of the problems is diagnosed and treated.

Cataracts can develop in the eyes if treatment is delayed for too long.

Later problems can include **specific speech defects** and eventual **ovarian failure** in a high proportion of girls with galactosemia.

Seizures can occur.

Treatment is by exclusion of all milk and milk products from the diet. If this change in diet occurs within the first week or two of life, damage to the liver, brain, and eyes can be avoided. If diagnosis has been delayed, and milk has been given for some weeks, jaundice, vomiting, and loss of weight will become a grave problem, although these symptoms will improve once milk has been removed from the child's diet. Regrettably, however, cataract formation, mental retardation, and possible liver damage can be permanent.

Avoidance of all milk products must be maintained throughout life. A number of commercial replacements, such as soybean products and casein hydrolysates, are available to satisfy the nutritional requirements of the baby. Normal physical growth can readily be maintained on these products.

MANAGEMENT IMPLICATIONS

Early and adequate treatment of **infection** in the early days of life is of vital importance if the child is to survive. Special intensive care facilities may be needed for the babies that are very sick.

The **dietary aspect** of galactosemia is the main problem to be faced once the baby has survived the first few traumatic weeks of life. A dietitian's advice on suitable foods with which to replace galactose in the diet is a necessity for parents and other care givers. As the child matures, it is somewhat easier for him/her to avoid milk products, although the child may be under pressure from peers to eat or drink what they are eating or drinking. It must be explained carefully to the child, and to her/his immediate friends, that this course of action will cause harm.

Speech defects do seem to be more commonly found in children with galactosemia than in the general childhood population, expressive speech being most commonly affected. The help of a speech therapist is necessary under these circumstances to ensure that the child learns to speak understandably.

Any possibility of **mental handicap** must be carefully assessed. Routine developmental tests should pick up delays in any of the parameters tested. In this context, the speech delay common in this condition must be remembered. Early help with various skills in which the child has been found to be behind will be valuable. Teachers specializing in assisting preschool children can be especially helpful. When school age comes around, the type of school most suited to the child's abilities will need to be determined. Special schooling, or a unit with special resources, may be necessary for some children with galactosemia.

When reproductive age is reached, there may be **fertility problems.** Females with galactosemia not infrequently have ovarian failure, which renders them infertile. If pregnancy is achieved, genetic counseling and appropriate testing during the pregnancy are advisable.

Seizures are not usual, but, if present, they will need to be treated with the appropriate anticonvulsant medicine. Regular monitoring of any such drug regime must also be undertaken.

THE FUTURE

If the exclusion of milk and milk products from the diet begins early in the newborn period and continues throughout life, there will be few problems—apart from, of course, the nuisance of dietary restrictions.

Communication problems can persist into adult life in spite of appropriate therapy. Therefore, when career choices have to be made, it is wisest to avoid any career relying heavily on verbal communication. Infertility may also cause heartache.

SELF-HELP GROUPS

Parents of Galactosemic Children, Inc.
2148 Bryton Drive
Powell, OH 43065
http://www.galactosemia.org

American Liver Foundation
1425 Pompton Avenue
Cedar Grove, NJ 07009
800-223-0179
http://www.gastro.com/liverpg/galactos.htm

Alliance of Genetic Support Groups
4301 Connecticut Avenue, N.W., Suite 404
Washington, DC 20008-2304
202-966-5557 or 800-336-4363
email: info@geneticalliance.org

Gaucher Disease

ALTERNATIVE NAMES

Glucosylcerebroside lipidosis; familial splenic anemia.

INCIDENCE

There are three main types of Gaucher disease, but type 1 is by far the most common, and accounts for 90% of the cases. It will be the type discussed here. (Types 2 and 3 have central nervous system and pulmonary involvement as major features. Life expectancy beyond early life is poor in these two types.)

Gaucher disease is one of the "storage" diseases. In these diseases, certain specific substances are stored to excess in the body, and it is this condition that accounts for the signs and symptoms of each specific disease. In all cases of storage disease, lack of specific enzymes that normally break down the excessive substances is the basic cause of the problems. Gaucher disease is one of a large group of lyosomal storage disorders.

Gaucher disease is not common—figures of 1 in 100,000 people have been quoted, but in Ashkenazi Jews, the incidence is reported as being as high as 1 in 600. The carrier rate in that particular group of people is thought to be as high as 1 in 25. The sexes are equally affected.

Chorionic villus sampling and/or amniocentesis can detect this disease prenatally.

CAUSATION

Gaucher disease is inherited as an autosomal recessive characteristic. The gene concerned has been mapped to chromosome 1. The basic fault is a deficiency of the enzyme *glucocerebrosidase.*

CHARACTERISTICS

The typical features of Gaucher disease can occur at any time during childhood or early adult life; signs and symptoms can occur as early as one year of age.

The first obvious sign is often an **enlarged abdomen,** caused by an increase in the size of both the liver and the spleen, which are storing the excess of the unmetabolized lysosomal substances. At times, liver enlargement can give rise to **abdominal pain.** As the spleen—the organ situated high in the abdomen under the left lower ribs and concerned with the proper function of blood cells—enlarges, hematological effects occur.

A diminution in the red cells available to perform their oxygen-carrying function can cause **anemia.** General feelings of malaise and fatigue follow when anemia becomes severe.

Small hemorrhages into the skin and easy **bruising** can occur due to faulty clotting mechanisms. **Nose bleeds** can also become a problem.

Bone pain and **fractures** of bones can occur as the disease progresses. Such bone problems are caused by infiltration of the lyso-somal substances, which in turn are due to the basic enzyme deficiency.

MANAGEMENT IMPLICATIONS

As the course of this condition is so variable, not every child will require the treatment outlined. Routine medical checks and parental concern will identify needs as they arise.

Splenectomy—removal of the spleen, either completely or partially—may become necessary if anemia and / or hemorrhages become too much of a problem. This operation, of course, must only be undertaken with the full cooperation of the pediatrician, the surgeon, and the hematology department.

Any **fractures** must be treated quickly and adequately. Orthopedic advice may be necessary for deformities that can result from the effects on the bone of the lysosomal deposits. (In cases of suspected child abuse, the pathological nature of fractures must always be remembered in a child with Gaucher disease.)

Bone pain will usually decrease if the affected limb is immobilized for a short period of time.

Schooling can be in a mainstream facility, but teachers should be aware of their pupil's inherited condition. Contact sports must be avoided, given both the increased likelihood of fractures and the (remote) possibility that an enlarged spleen will rupture.

Enzyme replacement and **bone marrow transplantation** are options that are currently being explored.

THE FUTURE

Life expectancy is not usually reduced for people with the above type of Gaucher disease. Genetic counseling is indicated before pregnancy is contemplated.

Fractures of the neck of the femur are more likely to occur in older people with this condition. Hip replacement may be necessary in early adult life due to this complication of Gaucher disease.

SELF-HELP GROUP

National Gaucher Foundation
11140 Rockville Pike, Suite 350
Rockville, MD 20852-3106
800-925-8885 or 301-816-1515
http://www.gaucherdisease.org
email: ngf@gaucherdisease.org

Goldenhar Syndrome

ALTERNATIVE NAMES

Goldenhar–Gorlin syndrome; ocular-auriculo-vertebral anomaly; first and second branchial arch syndrome.

INCIDENCE

Studies on the incidence of this syndrome have only been recorded in the USA. In the American midwest, one report observed an incidence of 1 in every 5,600 live births. A further study reported an incidence of 1 in every 26,000 live births in the USA. There appears to be a slightly higher incidence of this syndrome in boys than in girls.

CAUSATION

Patterns of inheritance seem to vary, and both an autosomal dominant and an autosomal recessive inheritance appear to be possible. The effects of the manifestations of this syndrome vary greatly, even within the same family. This variance makes accurate diagnosis, as well as the analysis of inheritance patterns, difficult.

Prenatal ultrasound examination may be able to detect ear abnormalities if they are present and severe. Other skeletal abnormalities, including the small lower jaw, may also be visualized through ultrasound.

CHARACTERISTICS

Ears: Abnormalities in the anatomy of both the external and the middle ear are among the most obvious, and important, features. The size and shape of the external ear varies greatly, ranging from virtually no external ear at all to a much misshapen pinna. Such deformities can occur in one or both ears. Ossicles, those tiny bones of the middle ear that are vital for normal hearing, can also be tiny or misshapen. If these ossicles are small and/or misshapen, sound will not be conducted properly to the nerves of hearing, and a conductive hearing loss will occur.

In conjunction with these abnormalities in the ear, the facial nerve can occasionally run an unusual course. The eustachian tube, linking the middle ear to the back of the throat, is also sometimes malformed. These defects can all add to the hearing problem.

Asymmetry of the face is another feature affecting the majority of the babies born with this syndrome. The asymmetry becomes more evident as the baby matures, and by the age of around four years, the unusual shape of the child's face is very obvious.

Cleft palate, with occasionally a coexistent cleft lip, can add to the unusual facial features at birth.

A **small, receding chin** can be a characteristic. If this feature is present, difficulties with feeding can be worrying in the early days of life.

Eyes may be small, with a narrowing of the actual eyelids that makes the eyes appear even smaller. About one-third of children with Goldenhar syndrome have pinkish-yellowish growths, often containing much fatty tissue, associated with their eyes. These growths can grow to be as large as 10 millimeters in diameter. If they reach this size, vision can become obscured.

A wide range of **skeletal abnormalities** can be present, varying from unusually shaped vertebrae, which will eventually give rise to scoliosis, to abnormalities in the forearm and thumbs. (These latter features are reminiscent of the abnormalities seen in both CHARGE and VATER associations, which also show defects in the forearm region. There is, however, no connection between these conditions and Goldenhar syndrome.)

Heart defects occur with greater frequency than in other babies. Reports as to the incidence of this type of abnormality varies. Some authorities put the incidence as high as 58% of babies born with Goldenhar syndrome. Ventricular septal defects are reported to be one of the most common of these heart abnormalities.

In a few children with this syndrome, there may be some degree of **mental retardation.**

Some children with very deformed faces can have severe **emotional problems.**

MANAGEMENT IMPLICATIONS

In the early days of life, **feeding** can be a problem if the baby has a tiny lower jaw (cf. Pierre–Robin syndrome). When present, a cleft palate, with or without an associated cleft lip, will add to the feeding difficulties. Tube feeding may be necessary in the early days to ensure adequate nutrition. The most severe cases can need surgical intervention to allow feedings to be given directly into the stomach. The unusual facial features can also lead to **breathing difficulties,** especially during sleep. A tiny lower jaw can allow the tongue to fall back into the throat, thereby obstructing breathing. Babies should be put to sleep on their sides to avoid this potential problem.

Hearing loss must also be diagnosed and fully assessed as early in life as possible to minimize the risk of delayed speech. The maximum age for the acquisition of speech and language is usually between one and two years. Before this time, the baby gathers information regarding various sound patterns by listening, especially to his/her parents. Any loss of hearing at either of these important stages can delay speech. Once the hearing loss is diagnosed and treated as far as is possible, **speech therapy** is valuable and often necessary for clear, understandable speech. In addition to communication problems due to hearing disabilities, children with Goldenhar syndrome can have difficulties articulating their words due to their unusual facial features. Speech therapists have many methods of overcoming all these problems.

Eyes: if the typical growths are present in the eye region, they should be removed before their increasing size further precludes vision. Unfortunately, vision can also be adversely affected after this removal by the scar tissue that inevitably forms following the operation.

If the child has a **cleft palate,** it will need surgical repair. Surgery may also be needed for other facial asymmetries if they are severe and amenable to this form of treatment.

Dental care is important following the eruption of the teeth. Due to the asymmetry of the face, teeth will not always meet together properly, so orthodontic care will be necessary.

Heart defects, if present, will need assessment and possibly treatment, depending on the type of defect and its effects on the child.

Mental abilities will need to be checked by routine developmental assessment at regular intervals, and assessment must be continued during the school years. Problems in any specific areas can thus be isolated and appropriate help given.

Emotional problems can arise, particularly during the adolescent years, if the facial disfigurement is very marked. Sensitive counseling and support from relatives and friends should reduce the impact of such problems to a minimum. Joining a group of similarly affected people can also do much to help.

THE FUTURE

Life span is not restricted unless heart defects are severe or not amenable to treatment.

Career choices may be limited if there is any substantial hearing loss. Facial disfigurement may make careers in the public eye difficult.

Genetic counseling when pregnancy is being considered is advisable.

SELF-HELP GROUPS

Goldenhar Syndrome Research and Information Fund
P.O. Box 61643
St. Petersburg, FL 33714
813-522-5772
email: 76232.633@compuserve.com

Goldenhar Parent Support Network
3619 Chicago Avenue
Minneapolis, MN 55407-2603
612-823-3529

Children's Craniofacial Association
P.O. Box 280297
Dallas, TX 75228
800-535-3643 or 972-994-9902
email: CHAR SMITH@prodigy.net

Gorlin Syndrome

Gorlin–Goltz Syndrome; basal cell nevus syndrome.

INCIDENCE

The exact incidence is unrecorded, and it is difficult to identify the condition clinically until jaw cysts or skin cancers become apparent. Family histories often reveal other family members who have had similar problems during their lives. Both boys and girls can be affected.

HISTORY

Gorlin syndrome is a recently described syndrome that has relatively few specific characteristics. Its importance lies in the inherited predisposition that children with the syndrome have to develop skin cancers and multiple cysts in the jaws.

CAUSATION

The gene defect for Gorlin syndrome is found on chromosome 9. The condition is thought to be inherited in an autosomal dominant manner. Genetic analysis to determine whether or not other family members have the faulty gene is possible.

CHARACTERISTICS

The syndrome has few characteristics, although it has been reported that children with Gorlin syndrome are often tall and well built. Luxuriant hair growth with a low hair-line on the forehead has also been described.

The other main features are:

- The appearance of **basal cell cancers** anywhere on the body. These are localized cancers, and they rarely spread if they are removed surgically during the early stages of the disease. Any child with a persistent reddened skin lesion that does not heal, or at least improve, within a few weeks should seek medical advice.

- **Cysts** arising in the bones of the jaw. These are not usually malignant, but if they are not recognized and treated, they will continue to enlarge and give rise to pain as nerves and tooth roots in the jaw are compressed.

A further feature of Gorlin syndrome that can help with diagnosis is the tendency for **calcium deposits** to be laid down in various parts of the body. These deposits rarely give rise to any problem, but they can be noted as incidental findings on X-ray examinations.

MANAGEMENT IMPLICATIONS

Regular skin and jaw screening must be conducted so that skin cancers and/or jaw cysts can be found early. Parents need to be alerted to these possibilities—if experiences with other family members have not already educated them.

Regular **dental check-ups**—with a dentist who is informed of the family predisposition—will be necessary, especially if the child complains of pain in the jaw.

THE FUTURE

With careful screening and treatment of any abnormalities, a normal lifestyle is assured.

SELF-HELP GROUPS

There is no known group dedicated to Gorlin syndrome, but the following organizations may offer useful information:

Skin Cancer Foundation
P.O. Box 561
New York, NY 10156
800-SKIN-490
http://www.skincancer.org
email: info@skincancer.org

American Cancer Society
1599 Clifton Road, NE
Atlanta, GA 30329
800-ACS-2345
http://www2.cancer.org

Guillain–Barré Syndrome

ALTERNATIVE NAME
Acute inflammatory polyneuropathy.

INCIDENCE

The true incidence of Guillain–Barré syndrome is not known. There have been suggestions that the incidence in children has increased over the past two decades. The most common time for the condition to occur seems to be between the ages of four and ten, although Guillain–Barré syndrome is not unknown in babies or adults. Boys and girls appear to be equally affected.

CAUSATION

There has been much discussion over the years regarding the cause of Guillain–Barré syndrome. Because the condition frequently follows after a person has an acute infection, the syndrome may be due to the toxic effects of this original infection. Hypersensitivity to some substance or organism, or the re-activation of a latent virus, have been other suggestions as to the cause.

There is no inheritance pattern involved in Guillain–Barré syndrome.

CHARACTERISTICS

Guillain–Barré syndrome will often start with **tingling** in the hands and feet. Along with these sensations will go severe pains in the legs and tenderness when muscles are touched. This latter symptom is due to inflammation of the sensory nerves. The severity of all these symptoms can vary, ranging from acute pain to only intermittent tingling sensations.

Within a few days, legs will become markedly weak, and walking will be difficult. This weakness gradually extends up the body to the arms and, most serious of all, to the muscles involved with respiration. The young sufferer will feel generally unwell, and she/he may have a mild fever, although this symptom is often not a feature.

Symptoms will persist and may worsen for around a week or two, during which time the child is gravely ill. Admission to the hospital is necessary, and artificial ventilation may be needed to maintain breathing. Muscles around the face and throat can also become involved, making swallowing difficult or impossible.

Once this acute stage is over, recovery begins. This process is slow, and many months may pass before the young sufferer is well again and able to use weakened muscles fully. Recovery is usually complete, and only a very small minority of children are left with any residual weakness. If this weakness does occur, the disability is only minimal.

MANAGEMENT IMPLICATIONS

Acute stage: once the diagnosis has been made, admission to the hospital is urgently necessary. Intensive care facilities need to be readily available to ensure that respiration is maintained. There is no specific treatment available; the patient will rely on good nursing care, and ventilator support may become necessary.

Convalescence can be long, with paralyzed muscles only slowly returning to full use. During this time, children will need adequate rest, a good diet, and plenty of quiet activities available. In later stages of convalescence, schoolwork can be sent home so that too much schooling is not missed.

THE FUTURE

Guillain–Barré syndrome is a serious illness, but in the long-term, the outlook is good, with little or no permanent sequelae.

SELF-HELP GROUP

Guillain–Barré Syndrome International
P.O. Box 262
Wynnewood, PA 19096
610-667-0131
http://www.webmast.com/gbs
email: gbint@ix.netcom.com

Hemolytic Uremic Syndrome

INCIDENCE

This syndrome is rare, but it can arise in geographic clusters. There are two quite separate ways in which this syndrome can arise, one of which is inherited and the other occurring as the result of an infection with a specific bacteria, E. Coli 0157.

The exact occurrence is not known, but the annual incidence is thought to range from 1 to 30 in every 100,000 persons. Children are the primary age group affected. A higher incidence of the syndrome is seen during the warmer months of the year.

CAUSATION

The hereditary form of this syndrome arises as either an autosomal dominant or an autosomal recessive condition. This inherited causative factor is thought to account for only a small number (about 5%) of the known cases.

Other children can suffer from hemolytic uremic syndrome as a result of a previous acute gastrointestinal illness. It can be difficult to distinguish the hereditary form of this syndrome from the acquired type, but there are two specific features that can point to one or other of the causative factors. First, in the acquired form of hemolytic uremic syndrome, symptoms of severe gastroenteritis (bloody diarrhea, vomiting, and a reduction in the amount of urine) are the early features of the condition. In the case of the inherited form, there is rarely any such preceding gastric upset—the characteristic features arise "out of the blue." Second, with the acquired type, other family members may become sick with a similar illness within days or weeks of the first sufferer's illness, thus pointing to an infectious cause. A toxin produced by the bacteria E. Coli 0157 is considered the cause of this syndrome. The bacteria can be food-borne or passed from person to person if good hygiene is not practiced. With the inherited form, the illness can appear in an affected individual anytime from infancy to about 14 years of age.

Hemolytic uremic syndrome can affect children at any age from a few months onward, but incidence is highest in children under the age of five years.

Reservoirs of E.Coli are found in the intestines of cattle—therefore, meat and unpasteurized milk from such animals can be a source of infection. Insufficiently washed vegetables, such as lettuce, can also harbor the bacteria.

CHARACTERISTICS

After the acute gastrointestinal infection seen in cases of presumed infectious origin, the following features occur:

Anemia of a hemolytic type—the child will be pale and lethargic, feel unwell, and tire easily on the slightest exertion. Blood tests reveal that the red blood cells are distorted and fragmented, causing them to lose much of their contained hemoglobin (the oxygen-carrying substance in the red blood cells). The platelet count is also often extremely low. (Platelets are intimately concerned with the clotting of the blood.) Hemorrhages under the skin can arise as a result of these blood changes. Bloody diarrhea is a relatively constant feature of infection with E. Coli.

Renal failure can rapidly develop. Urine output may be much reduced, or there may be no urination at all. The urine that is produced is bloodstained. The child is acutely and seriously ill, with perhaps a very elevated blood pressure and cardiac failure. He/she will be restless and confused, and seizures can occur. Death can result during this very serious acute phase of the illness.

The **central nervous system, heart, lungs** and **pancreas** can also be affected.

(The pathology behind these serious events is thought to be damage to walls of the tiny blood vessels inside the kidneys and/or other organs, which in turn injures the blood cells. A defect in the metabolism of a specific chemical, prostacyclin, has been suggested to be the prime cause of hemolytic uremic syndrome.)

Following the acute illness, damage to the central nervous system (probably as a result of the seizures that can occur), may happen, resulting in a residual **learning disability.** Such a disability does not always occur, but it must be remembered as a possibility. A recurrence of the acute illness can occur in some children at a later date. This particular occurrence is thought only to happen in those people who suffer from the hemolytic uremic syndrome that arises as a recessively inherited characteristic.

Treatment includes dialysis to combat the acute renal failure. A blood transfusion will be necessary to treat the hemolytic anemia. This transfusion must be given with care so as not to overload the circulation, with the concomitant damaged renal output, with fluid.

Chronic renal failure may be the unfortunate end result if the acute stage of the disease is survived. The affected person may require repeated hemodialysis or continuous peritoneal dialysis. Kidney transplantation is the best long-term option.

MANAGEMENT IMPLICATIONS

A person in the **acute** stage of hemolytic uremic syndrome will need intensive care facilities in the hospital to combat renal failure and possible hypertension and cardiac failure. Any succeeding recurrences of the condition must also to be treated in a similar way.

Continuous ambulatory peritoneal dialysis may be the best way to treat a child with chronic renal failure following acute illness while he/she is awaiting renal transplantation. Children accept this necessary treatment surprisingly well and become adept at coping with their unusual excretory process.

Learning disability following from the acute illness must be recognized and subjected to detailed assessment. A few children may require special educational facilities; in those cases, ongoing assessment and help must be given.

PREVENTION

Prevention rests with public health measures monitoring hygiene practices throughout the food chain. The strictest hygiene practices should be followed in all food handling situations, especially in the home.

THE FUTURE

The outlook for persons with the inherited form of hemolytic uremic syndrome is not good. In one report, between 70 and 90% of the persons with the inherited form died as a result of their illness, and 6% of the survivors were in chronic renal failure. Further attacks of acute illness may also occur.

Survivors of the acquired type may also suffer from chronic renal failure, or they may make a complete recovery. It is important that any child who has suffered such an infectious episode receives long-term medical follow-up.

Career prospects will depend on the amount of residual handicap. Life expectancy will also depend on the severity of the after-effects. Genetic counseling is indicated, particularly in those families in which more than one member has the condition.

SELF-HELP GROUP

Lois Joy Galler Foundation
734 Walt Whitman Road
Melville, NY 11747
516-673-3017
http://www.loisjoygaller.org

Hemophilia A

ALTERNATIVE NAMES

Classic hemophilia; factor 8 deficiency.

INCIDENCE

The incidence of this well-known inherited condition is 1 in every 10,000 live male births (only boys are affected, due to the mode of inheritance). All races can be affected.

Hemophilia is a term used to describe a number of blood disorders, all of which have clotting problems as their basic defect. There are a number of "factors" associated with the clotting mechanism of the blood. In hemophilia A specifically, it is factor 8 that is deficient. Other factors are involved in the clotting disorders of other similar diseases, such as Christmas disease and Von Willebrand disease.

HISTORY

Hemophilia has been known for many years, and it is well documented in history. Effective treatment was not available until the early 1960s. Prior to that decade, hemophilia was often fatal in childhood, or it led to much disability and a restricted lifestyle.

CAUSATION

Hemophilia A has an X-linked recessive inheritance. There is an abnormal factor 8 molecule in sufferers from this condition, and this factor leads to the abnormal clotting mechanism. Between one-fifth and one-third of all cases are thought to arise sporadically as new mutations. The disease can be mild, moderate, or severe. It is thought that each of these three manifestations of the disease may have a distinctive type of genetic inheritance. About one-half of all known cases of classic hemophilia have the severe form of the disease. About 80% of sufferers have a positive family history of hemophilia.

The condition can be diagnosed prenatally by fetoscopy.

CHARACTERISTICS

All the features of hemophilia are entirely due to the defective clotting mechanism. The condition can be diagnosed at birth. Excessive bleeding from the umbilical cord can be the first clue as to the possibility of a bleeding disorder.

In severely affected boys, **hemorrhages** into joints are common. Such hemorrhages can occur following only minimal trauma, or they may result from nothing more than the usual vigorous movements of joints common to all active children. Hips, knees, and ankles can all be affected, as can wrists and elbows. This condition leads to **painful, swollen joints,** the excess blood inside the capsules of the joints causing the pain. Appropriate treatment must be given early to avoid damage to, and the eventual destruction of, the affected joints. Before the advent of specific treatment, frequent hemorrhagic incidents inevitably resulted in grossly deformed joints caused by degenerative arthritis. This affliction was especially evident in weight-bearing joints such as hips and knees.

Bruising in soft tissues all over the body is commonly seen in hemophiliac boys. Again, this damage results from only minor bumps.

In young children, bleeding from minor injuries to the **tongue** and **lips** is common. During the early days of learning to walk, falls are common and are often associated with damage to the mouth region. Inadvertent biting of the tongue is also common when a child is learning to cope with solid food. These everyday mishaps can lead to severe hemorrhages in the boy with hemophilia.

Bumps on the **head** are also very common during the growing years, and they can result in disastrous bleeding into the brain in hemophiliac boys unless rapid treatment is given. Such injuries are one of the major causes of death in the young child with hemophilia.

In cases of suspected child abuse, the possibility of hemophilia—if not already known—must be considered as an alternative explanation for the child's injuries.

Less severely affected children will not be so vulnerable to minor injury. It is only when surgery (for example, a tonsillectomy or other relatively minor procedure) is undertaken that the clotting defect is a problem. Serious accidents will also result in severe bleeding.

Hemophiliac boys are especially susceptible to infection with **hepatitis B,** which can lead to progressive, potentially fatal liver disease. As soon as the diagnosis of hemophilia is made, the boy should be immunized against hepatitis B.

Treatment consists of giving factor 8. Prompt infusion of this compound will limit the damage done by bleeding into joints. As soon as the bleeding occurs, the treatment must be given. Some boys with hemophilia will develop a specific "inhibitor," or immunity, to routine treatment. Subsequent hemorrhagic events will then need to be treated at a specialized hematology department.

Some years ago, many blood products used to treat hemophiliac patients were, regrettably, contaminated with HIV, and a number of sufferers have succumbed to AIDS as a result. Heat-treated products, which render HIV noninfectious, are now used for treatment.

MANAGEMENT IMPLICATIONS

It can be difficult to strike the correct balance between overprotection and lack of restraint when dealing with a boy with hemophilia. Parents will feel that they must avoid even the slightest injury to their son. On the other hand, the child must be allowed to explore and investigate his environment as part of the growing process. It is all too easy for the boy with hemophilia to develop **emotional problems** as he tries to deal with his genetic inheritance. Support and advice from doctors, nurses, and other professionals experienced in the handling of children with hemophilia is important.

Parents become very experienced during the early years in assessing the significance of any injury, and they will also become adept at giving appropriate treatment.

Schooling will obviously present greater risks to the hemophiliac child. Teachers must be fully conversant with the action to be taken if a fall or other injury results in bleeding into a joint or other tissues. The telephone number of the hematologist responsible for the treatment of the child should be available in school. If in any doubt exists as to the action to be taken following an injury, advice can be obtained from this source.

Contact sports and other violent physical activities must not be part of the curriculum for the hemophiliac boy.

Education has an important part to play in the future career of a boy with this condition. Manual work cannot be contemplated, so intellectual pursuits and careers are of vital importance.

Care should also be taken in the use of aspirin in hemophiliac boys.

VON WILLEBRAND DISEASE (PSEUDO-HEMOPHILIA)

Like hemophilia A, this condition has a relative deficiency in factor 8. Unlike hemophilia A, Von Willebrand disease can affect both boys and girls, as the inheritance pattern is either an autosomal dominant or an autosomal recessive.

Symptoms of bleeding are much less in Von Willebrand disease than in hemophilia A. Nevertheless, epistaxis (nosebleed) is common, and bruising on minimal injury can result. For girls, excessive menstrual flow can be a problem resulting in much discomfort and possibly anemia. Excessive bleeding following surgery can be a problem for both male and female sufferers.

Treatment consists of giving cryoprecipitate factor 8. Immunization against hepatitis B is also a wise precaution.

Following childbirth, care must be taken to control bleeding in women with Von Willebrand disease.

THE FUTURE

With adequate quick treatment of bleeding episodes, the outlook is good nowadays for hemophiliac boys. Careers that include physical activities and body-contact sports must be avoided.

SELF-HELP GROUP

World Federation of Hemophilia
1425 René Lévesque Boulevard West, Suite 1010
Montreal, Quebec H3G 1T7
Canada
514-875-7944
http://www.wfh.org
email: wfh@wfh.org

Holt–Oram Syndrome

Heart–Hand syndrome.

INCIDENCE

Holt–Oram syndrome is an uncommon syndrome, which has neverthe-less been reported worldwide in many different populations. Both boys and girls can be affected. Ultrasound scanning in pregnancy can detect some of the more severe limb deformities.

HISTORY

This syndrome was first described by Drs. Holt and Oram in the early 1960s. It is interesting to note that the abnormalities associated with the syndrome are similar to those that occurred in the babies of women who took thalidomide for the relief of morning sickness in the early weeks of pregnancy. It is thought that the abnormal gene in Holt–Oram syndrome is probably active at roughly the same stage in pregnancy when women might consume thalidomide.

CAUSATION

This condition is inherited as an autosomal dominant, but with variable expression. For example, a severely affected parent may have a less affected child, or vice versa. Occasionally, the condition occurs sporadi-cally.

CHARACTERISTICS

As the alternative name for Holt–Oram syndrome suggests, there are two major features to this condition:

Congenital heart disease is the most serious aspect of the syn-drome, but this disease is usually amenable to corrective surgery. The most common abnormality is an atrial septal defect (an opening between the two upper [collecting] chambers of the heart). A ventricular septal defect (an opening between the two lower [pumping] chambers of the heart) can also occur. Other congenital cardiac conditions can occur, such as a patent ductus or transposition of the great arteries.

Skeletal features of the syndrome are restricted to the upper limbs—the lower limbs are not involved at all. The characteristics of the **skeletal abnormalities** can vary from very short forearms to a complete absence of these limbs. The thumb is frequently involved; it can be small and underdeveloped, or it can have an extra bone. Occasionally, there are only 3 fingers present. Shoulders and collarbones can also be affected, making shoulders narrow with a downward slant.

There are no other abnormalities associated with this syndrome, and intellectual abilities are normal.

MANAGEMENT IMPLICATIONS

The **heart abnormalities** will need corrective surgery as soon as the baby is mature enough to withstand the operative procedure. Depending on the type of defect, the outcome is generally good, and a normal life can be led following recovery.

The impact of the **skeletal abnormalities** will depend on their type and severity. Severe difficulties will be experienced throughout life when forearms are absent or very short; a lack of digits or an unusually shaped thumb will also cause considerable problems. Training in self-help skills, writing, and drawing will need specialized and ongoing.

Milder degrees of abnormality will probably affect functional skills very little, Children are especially good at adapting to such difficulties.

THE FUTURE

The future will depend on the type and degree of disability of both heart and limb. The lifestyle and life span of persons who are minimally affected are normal.

SELF-HELP GROUPS

There are no known organizations in the United States dedicated specifically to Holt–Oram syndrome, but the following groups may offer assistance:

Congenital Heart Anomalies, Support, Education, and Resources
2112 North Wilkins Road
Swanton, OH 43558
419-825-5575
http://www.csun.edu/~hfmth006/chaser/
email: myer106w@wonder.em.cdc.gov or chaser@compuserve.com

Superkids, Inc.
60 Clyde Street
Newton, MA 02460-2250
http://www.super-kids.org

Holt-Oram Syndrome Support Group
21 Forth Road, Rivers Estate
Redcar, Cleveland, TS10- 1PN
United Kingdom
164-248-5379
http://www.btinternet.com/~holt.oram/holt.oram.htm
email: Holt.Oram@btinternet.com

Homocystinuria

Homocystinuria is a rare metabolic disease. As with other metabolic conditions, knowledge about the biochemical nature of the problem has vastly increased over the past decade. As a result of the programs screening newborn babies in most parts of the world, it has been found that Ireland appears to have one of the highest incidences of homocystinuria. In that country, 1 in 60,000 babies is likely to be affected, whereas the number of babies in Japan with this particular metabolic problem has been estimated to be as low as 1 in 146,000. Both boys and girls can be affected.

CAUSATION

Homocystinuria is inherited as an autosomal recessive condition.

CHARACTERISTICS

Homocystinuria is a defect in the enzyme metabolism of specific amino acids—homocystine and methionine. Excess homocystine is excreted in the urine, and both homocystine and methionine can be found in excess in the plasma.

These two facts form the basis of the biochemical diagnosis and also result in the following features.

Skeletal system: children with homocystinuria are usually tall with long, slender fingers. (This characteristic, together with the similar eye problems, resemble the features found in Marfan syndrome.) Scoliosis may also be present, as well as knock-knees and chest deformities.

Eyes are commonly affected in homocystinuria, dislocation of the lens being the most common abnormality. Myopia is also common, and glaucoma and retinal detachment are further complications that can occur later in life. Appropriate treatment when, and if, these complications occur can reduce the incidence of severe visual problems.

Blood system: effects on the vascular system are the most worrying aspects of homocystinuria. Thromboses occur with greater frequency than normal, and they can occur anywhere in the body—brain, heart, or eyes, for example. Symptoms will occur in relationship to the part of the vascular system that is affected. (Due to the danger of thromboses, venipuncture and surgical procedures should be avoided if at all possible, or certainly undertaken with great care.) This abnormal clotting can occur at any time of life, including infancy and childhood. The exact mechanism of this phenomenon is not fully understood.

Central nervous system: most homocystinuria sufferers have normal mental abilities, but a minority show mild to moderate mental retardation. Early treatment does seem to help mitigate this development. If thrombosis has occurred in the brain, it may have a deleterious effect on mental abilities as well as the physical neurological signs. Seizures can also occur, although this problem is comparatively rare, and, again, can be helped by appropriate treatment.

MANAGEMENT IMPLICATIONS

In some cases of homocystinuria, treatment with vitamin B6 (pyridoxine) improves many features of the disease. It is of vital importance that doctors determine early whether the individual is susceptible to treatment with pyridoxine so that various manifestations of the condition can be alleviated. The vitamin is given on a regular basis, and levels of the relevant amino acids in the blood are measured regularly. If these levels approach normal limits, treatment is continued throughout life, with, of course, regular monitoring.

Folic acid supplements also appear to be necessary in some people with homocystinuria. This supplement maximizes the good effects of the vitamin B6. A diet low in methionine can also be valuable, and the help of a dietitian is of great value under these circumstances.

Eyes: visual acuity must be assessed regularly and corrective lenses prescribed for any refractive error found. The increased possibility of glaucoma and retinal detachment must also be borne in mind.

Vascular system: any thrombotic episodes, with the possible damaging sequelae, must be managed medically as they occur.

Central nervous system: children should receive regular developmental checks, with monitoring continuing when school age is reached. Appropriate schooling can then be arranged should any problems be found. Checking of intellectual abilities after any central nervous system thrombotic episodes is also advisable.

THE FUTURE

With appropriate early treatment in the vitamin B6–responsive type of homocystinuria, the outlook is good, and life expectancy is normal. Individuals that do not respond to vitamin B6 will have to rely on dietary measures as the sole form of available treatment. Under these circumstances, life-threatening thromboses are more likely to occur, but research is showing that early dietary restrictions, conscientiously adhered to throughout life, do improve the outlook.

Due to the increased risk of thrombosis, the use of oral contraceptives is not recommended.

SELF-HELP GROUP

Alliance of Genetic Support Groups
4301 Connecticut Avenue, N.W., Suite 404
Washington, DC 20008-2304
202-966-5557 or 800-336-4363
http://www.geneticalliance.org
email: info@geneticalliance.org

Hunter Syndrome

ALTERNATIVE NAME

Mucopolysaccharidosis 2.

INCIDENCE

Hunter syndrome is an example of a defect in the metabolism of the complex sugars, the mucopolysaccharides. There are a number of syndromes in this group, and in each syndrome, there is lack of a specific enzyme that controls the metabolism of these nutrients. (Other syndromes in this group include Hurler syndrome, Morquio syndrome, and Sanfilippo syndrome.) Around 1 baby in 100,000 live births exhibits Hunter syndrome. Due to the mode of inheritance of Hunter syndrome, only boys have been known to be affected. All races of the world appear to be affected.

HISTORY

Until relatively recently, only seven mucopolysaccharide syndromes had been described—each due to a different enzyme defect. Recently however, 11 variants have been found, each with defective metabolism of a complex sugar. It is possible that further similar enzyme defects can occur.

CAUSATION

Hunter syndrome is inherited in an X-linked recessive way, so no girls are seen with Hunter syndrome. Mothers carrying the characteristics can pass them onto their sons. The enzyme involved in Hunter syndrome is a complicated one known as iduronate sulphatase. Due to the deficiency of this enzyme, mucopolysaccharides accumulate in the organs and tissues of the body, where these complex sugars give rise to the typical signs and symptoms of the syndrome.

Hunter syndrome can be detected at around the ninth week of pregnancy by chorionic villus sampling techniques.

CHARACTERISTICS

There are two types of Hunter syndrome—one of which is milder and runs a less progressively downhill course than the more severe type.

These two types can be distinguished biochemically by the complex sugar that is excreted in the urine. It is the accumulation of the specific sugar in the organs and tissues that gives rise to the following characteristics.

Boys with Hunter syndrome appear to have no problems at birth. They grow normally and pass all their developmental milestones at the proper time. During these early days, the only noticeable problem can be noisy breathing, which is frequently associated with a blocked and runny nose. As this symptom is often part of normal childhood, it does not alert anyone to other possible problems. Head circumference measurements are within the upper limits of normal during these early years.

Umbilical, or inguinal, **hernias** are more frequently seen in babies who are subsequently found to have Hunter syndrome than is usual. Once again, because boys who do not have Hunter syndrome can also have these weaknesses in the abdominal wall, that symptom does not usually cause suspicions that the syndrome may be a concern.

From around two years of age onward, there is an obvious coarsening of the **facial features.** The boy's neck will be short, and his erupting teeth will be widely spaced. Over the succeeding months, these features are combined with a slowing down of the growth rate.

Joints can become stiff and the body is often covered with fine, downy **hair.**

At this time, the **liver** and **spleen** become enlarged as a direct result of the accumulation of mucopolysaccharides in those organs. The enlargement can be a factor in the onset—or recurrence—of the umbilical hernia.

Mentally, children with the mild form of Hunter syndrome are of normal intelligence or only very mildly handicapped. Unfortunately, with the severe form, mental handicap is greater and will be obvious by around the age of eight to ten years.

As the boy matures, deposits of mucopolysaccharides can be found in many organs of the body—heart valves, coronary arteries, meninges, and joints all being possibly included. One, or more, of these complications can result in potentially fatal illnesses. For instance, damage to heart valves and/or coronary arteries can give rise to heart failure or, in the case of a blocked coronary artery, sudden death.

This clinical picture is very similar to that seen in the other muco-polysaccharidoses, although the basic genetic and biochemical faults are different.

MANAGEMENT IMPLICATIONS

There is, regrettably, no curative treatment for Hunter syndrome. Parents need sensitive counseling about the future of their son, it being important to emphasize the help that can be given to make life as normal as possible for their child—and themselves.

Hernia: if this weakness of the abdominal wall is present, it must be surgically corrected. There is, however, a high likelihood of recurrence, as further accumulations of mucopolysaccharides can increase the pressure inside the abdominal wall and push the contents into weakened areas.

Hearing must be checked on a regular basis. Distraction tests suitable to the mental age of the boy will need to be done. Pure-tone audiometry is a further option, with evoked responses as a further aid to diagnosis where necessary. Deafness is common, and hearing aids may be necessary later in childhood.

Contractures of joints, which can lead to grossly limited movement, can be kept to a minimum with physical therapy. Hydrotherapy is particularly valuable and soothing. Therapy should be ongoing, with parents involved in the treatment of their son as far as is possible. Surgery may sometimes be necessary to correct joint deformities.

Mental handicap in the severe type of Hunter syndrome means the child will need special education. Regular developmental checks are necessary to monitor all aspects of ongoing development in the boy with Hunter syndrome. The results of such monitoring are necessary when decisions are being made as to the suitability of special educational facilities.

With the milder type of Hunter syndrome, normal schooling is usually satisfactory.

THE FUTURE

Children with the severe type of Hunter syndrome often only survive into their mid-teens or twenties. Cardiac problems, or severe respiratory infection, are the usual cause of death in the early or mid-twenties.

Boys with the milder type of Hunter syndrome enjoy a longer life span, and men with the syndrome have been known to survive into their late sixties.

Children have been born to fathers with Hunter syndrome. Persons related to a boy with Hunter syndrome will need genetic counseling. Girls carrying the defective gene can be identified, and this identification is of crucial importance when pregnancy is being considered.

Gene therapy and enzyme replacement therapy are currently being researched.

SELF-HELP GROUP

National MPS Society, Inc.
102 Aspen Drive
Downington, PA 19335
610-942-0100
http://mpssociety.org
email: presmps@aol.com

Hurler Syndrome

ALTERNATIVE NAMES

Gargoylism; mucopolysaccharidosis 1-H.

INCIDENCE

Hurler syndrome is one of a group of diseases known as the mocu-polysaccharidoses. These conditions are all similar in that they all owe their characteristics to accumulations of mucopolysaccharides (complex sugars) in the tissues of the body. Enzymes necessary to the breakdown of these complex sugars are defective in these conditions. The enzyme responsible differs in each syndrome of this group.

All the mucopolysaccharide diseases differ clinically, genetically, and biochemically from each other. There are probably up to 11 different mucopolysaccharide abnormalities. (See Hunter syndrome, Morquio syndrome, and Sanfilippo syndrome. The remaining syndromes in this group are exceedingly rare.) Around 1 in 100,000 live births exhibit Hurler syndrome. The sexes are equally represented, and Hurler syndrome has been described in all races.

HISTORY

The mucopolysaccharidoses have been known for some time, but until recent years, the specific enzyme defect in each type had not been isolated. Classification has also been a problem in the past, but it has now been standardized.

CAUSATION

Hurler syndrome is caused by a genetic defect inherited as an autosomal recessive. The particular enzyme that is deficient in Hurler syndrome is alpha-L-iduronidase. This deficiency results in high levels of muco-polysaccharides being both excreted in the urine and deposited in the tissues.

Hurler syndrome can be detected prenatally by assay of the specific enzyme from chorionic villus sampling and also by amniocentesis.

CHARACTERISTICS

Children with Hurler syndrome appear to be normal at birth, although they may be very **large babies,** but from the early months of life onward the following features will appear.

Facial features will gradually become coarsened, with a depressed nasal bridge, large lips and tongue, and widely spaced teeth. Along with these features goes a persistently blocked and runny nose associated with noisy breathing.

Abdominally, a **large spleen and liver** may be felt and also seen. Many toddlers do normally have big abdomens due to the relatively large size of the liver at this age, but the child with Hurler syndrome will show this characteristic to excess. Also, the usual "slimming down" of the late preschool years will not occur; instead, the large abdomen will increase in size. By two years of age, there is frequently a large umbilical and/or inguinal hernia present, which is due to the increased pressure of abdominal organs enlarged by the accumulation of mucopolysaccharides.

Skeletal system: many joints become stiff and eventually lose much of their range of mobility altogether, unless steps are taken to correct this problem. The spine can become curved in both the upper and lower back regions; the former eventually giving rise to a grossly deformed chest. By two years of age, the child will be noticeably shorter than his/her contemporaries. Growth, which had been normal up to between six to 18 months, now proceeds only very slowly.

Eyes: the cornea becomes progressively clouded after the first few months of life. Vision eventually becomes very limited, due both to the corneal clouding and also to degenerative changes in the retina.

Mental retardation: as the child matures, deposits of mucopolysaccharides accumulate in the brain. This condition leads to a variable degree of mental retardation. Many children will lose some of the skills they have already learned.

Cardiac defects can arise at any time, due to deposits of mucopolysaccharides in the heart and coronary arteries. As the valves and walls of the coronary arteries become infiltrated, signs of heart failure can occur—breathlessness, swelling of lower limbs, or lassitude, for example.

There is another variant of Hurler syndrome, known as **Scheie syndrome** (mucopolysaccharidosis AS), which has a deficiency of the same enzyme as that which is deficient in Hurler syndrome. Characteristics are similar to those seen in Hurler syndrome, but they are much milder. The two syndromes have similar genetic inheritances.

MANAGEMENT IMPLICATIONS

Once the diagnosis has been made (by biochemical findings of reduced enzyme activity, elevation of specific mucopolysaccharides, and specific X-ray appearances in bones), plans will need to be made to care for a child who will have increasing mental and physical disabilities. Parents must be sensitively counseled as to the likely outcome of their child's genetic problem.

Umbilical and/or inguinal hernia will need surgery both to prevent the possibility of strangulation and for the child's comfort. Due to the continuing progressive accumulation of mucopolysaccharides, hernias may recur and need further treatment.

Stiff joints may also need surgical help, but physical therapy—particularly in warm water—will give symptomatic relief. Children enjoy this form of therapy very much.

Heart abnormalities need to be monitored closely by way of cardiac function. Surgical treatment may be found to be necessary, but it has not proved to be of long-lasting value due to the continuing nature of the underlying problem.

Mental retardation, visual difficulties, and **deafness,** all caused by progressive deposition of mucopolysaccharides, will mean that the child will eventually need special educational facilities. Frequent assessment of the possible deterioration of vision, hearing, or mental abilities is necessary, so that the child with Hurler syndrome can be cared for in an optimum environment. Methods of communication other than vision or hearing may need to be learned if usual methods of communication become a problem.

It is probable that the child with Hurler syndrome will eventually become wheelchair-bound. Special facilities in the child's home—and school—for toileting, bathing, and other activities will then be necessary.

THE FUTURE

Regrettably, because Hurler syndrome is a progressive disorder for which there is no cure at present, life expectancy is poor. Few children reach their teens. Death is caused by either pneumonia following the frequent respiratory illnesses or to heart failure.

Enzyme replacement therapy has been tried with limited success. At present, bone-marrow transplants are being evaluated, and research into gene therapy is continuing.

SELF-HELP GROUP

National MPS Society, Inc.
102 Aspen Drive
Downington, PA 19335
610-942-0100
http://mpssociety.org
email: presmps@aol.com

Hypertrophic Cardiomyopathy

ALTERNATIVE NAMES

Muscular subaortic stenosis; hypertrophic obstructive cardiomyopathy.

INCIDENCE

The exact incidence of this condition is not known, but is thought to be around 1 in 10,000. (It will probably never be possible to determine the exact incidence of hypertrophic cardiomyopathy. Many people are unaware that they have this cardiac abnormality because they never have any symptoms throughout life.) Hypertrophic cardiomyopathy may cause sudden death, even in young people, if the disease has not been recognized.

The condition has been reported from all over the world in people of all races. Both sexes are equally affected.

HISTORY

Hypertrophic cardiomyopathy was first recognized as a specific heart defect in the late 1950s.

CAUSATION

It is thought that this heart problem is inherited as an autosomal dominant condition. Once a diagnosis has been made in one family member, it is strongly recommended that first-degree relatives (parents, children, brothers, and sisters) be screened for the condition.

Reports of abnormalities in the genes on chromosome 14 in some families with hypertrophic cardiomyopathy have been received. Work is proceeding on the genetics of this condition.

CHARACTERISTICS

The basic abnormality in the hearts of people with hypertrophic cardiomyopathy is a **thickening in the wall of some part of the ventricles** (the "pumping" chambers of the heart)—usually the left—or in the septum dividing the two sides of the heart. When looked at under the microscope, the cells in the abnormal part of the heart appear randomly arranged instead of showing the symmetrical pattern seen in normal heart muscle. The overall effect of this abnormality is to reduce the pumping action of the heart. In addition to that problem, two further effects can occur:

- The "disarray" in the heart muscle can interfere with the normal electrical conducting mechanism controlling the **rhythm of the heart;**
- if the thickened part of the heart is high in the septum, it can interfere with the **action of the mitral valve.** This valve controls the blood flow between the left atrium and the left ventricle. (The atria of the heart are the two upper "collecting" chambers of the heart.)

Although this condition is probably present at birth in most cases, it is usually not until the teenage, or early adult years, that symptoms begin to occur. The reason why the condition becomes apparent—by the following symptoms—at this time is unclear.

Breathlessness accompanying any unusual exertion is often one of the first signs of problems. The teenager will not be able to keep up with peers in competitive games or cross-country running, for example. Alternatively, the sufferer may suddenly take a dislike to all forms of extra physical exercise, not liking to admit to becoming unduly breathless. (This symptom is so often correlated with advancing age!)

Chest pain can also be a warning sign. The pain is felt centrally in the chest and is often made worse by exercise, although it can occur when sitting quietly. The reason for this pain is probably a lack of oxygen sufficient for the thickened muscles to work properly.

Palpitations, in which the heart beat is irregular and, often most uncomfortably, at a fast rate, can be a symptom. At times, these irregularities can lead to feelings of **lightheadedness** and **dizziness,** and occasionally to a **loss of consciousness.** The risk of sudden death is greater in people with this condition than for those with completely normal hearts.

Endocarditis—an infection of the inner lining of the heart—is also a risk associated with this condition. Endocarditis is due to the greater ability of bacteria, present in the bloodstream in generalized infections, to stick to the roughened lining of the heart. This roughness is caused by the turbulence of the blood flow through the heart, which, in turn, is due to the thickened walls.

All the above symptoms must be more fully investigated to determine the true cause. If hypertrophic cardiomyopathy is suspected, further investigations will be necessary. (Only comparatively minor abnormalities associated with this syndrome can be heard through the stethoscope. For example, a stethoscope may detect a forceful heart beat, which is also transmitted to the pulses in wrist and neck, or, if the mitral valve is involved, a typical murmur may be heard.)

INVESTIGATIONS

An electrocardiogram will be necessary to show abnormal electrical signals due to the disorganization of the cardiac muscle. In a few people with hypertrophic cardiomyopathy, however, the EKG readings are normal. Under these latter circumstances, further investigations will be necessary if the physical symptoms suggest that hypertrophic cardiomyopathy is present; **echocardiography,** an ultrasound scan of the heart, will readily show the thickened muscles if these are present. Doppler ultrasound can also be used to produce images of the blood flow inside the heart and to measure the organ's filling capacity.

There are also a number of other investigations that may need to be done to obtain a clear picture of what is going on inside the heart:

- **Cardiac catheterization.** In this examination, a fine tube is passed into the heart from a blood vessel in the leg. The procedure is done under X-ray guidance. Through the test, pressures inside the heart can be measured and blood flow through the valves can be seen.
- **Continuous 24-hour EKG monitoring,** which is conducted by attaching a small EKG machine to the chest and placing a tape recorder in a small bag around the patient's waist. In this way, a continuous record of the heart's action can be obtained, showing the type and frequency of any arrhythmia.
- **Exercise tolerance tests.** Carefully graded exercise tests can also be a useful measure of heart function.

MANAGEMENT IMPLICATIONS

For many children and young people with this condition, its presence will not be known unless screening has taken place because another family member has been found to be suffering from hypertrophic cardiomyopathy. Even if the condition is known to be present, there may be no symptoms at all during early childhood. Still, care needs to be taken, without overprotecting the child.

Exercise should only be undertaken within the limits of cardiac function. Children who become breathless or otherwise distressed after exercise should not be allowed to take part in strenuous games or competitive sports.

Drugs, of various kinds, are only necessary if heart dysfunctions are present. A pediatrician and a cardiologist should cooperate to decide upon and closely monitor any drug regimen.

Antibiotics should be given prophylactically when any major dental work, such as the extraction of teeth, is undertaken. This precaution is intended to minimize the risk of endocarditis.

Diet. People with this condition are advised to follow a generally sensible diet designed to control excess weight, and to avoid smoking.

Overheating, such as in a hot bath, should be avoided.

THE FUTURE

Genetic counseling is advisable before pregnancy, so that the risk of the baby being affected by the condition can be estimated.

Pregnancy and labor can be entirely normal for the woman with hypertrophic cardiomyopathy. Pregnancy does, of course, impose an increased demand on the work of the heart, and some women may have symptoms due to their heart condition for the first time during pregnancy. Others who have had symptoms already may find these worsening. In these cases, specialist advice is necessary. Epidural anesthesia during labor is best avoided, as blood pressure can drop excessively.

SELF-HELP GROUP

Hypertrophic Cardiomyopathy Association
P.O. Box 306
Hibernia, NJ 07842
973-983-7429 (between 8 a.m. and 8 p.m., Eastern Standard Time)
email: LFAS1282@aol.com

Icthyosis

ALTERNATIVE NAMES

Icthyosis vulgaris; lamellar icthyosis; bullous icthyosis.

INCIDENCE

Icthyosis—meaning a persistent scaling of the skin—can occur in association with a number of syndromes and can also occur as a characteristic on
its own.

Syndromes that have these skin changes include the Sjogren–Larsson syndrome (in which spasticity and learning difficulties are associated
features); Refsum disease (in which abnormal concentrations of phytanic
acid in the tissues cause neurological problems and retinitis pigmentosa);
and Netherton syndrome (in which there is also alopecia and developmental delay).

The skin abnormalities are subdivided into a number of groups with
different types and degrees of severity.

The incidence of icthyosis vulgaris is thought to be as high as 1 in
250 births, but here again there is a wide range of types—from excessively
dry skin to a widespread scaling of many parts of the body surface.

Both boys and girls are equally affected.

CAUSATION

Icthyosis per se has an autosomal dominant inheritance. Pathologically,
there are either abnormalities in the shedding of dead epithelial cells,
abnormal keratinization, or changes in the lipid content of skin cells.

The skin changes are life-long, and they will need ongoing treatment.

CHARACTERISTICS

Icthyosis vulgaris—the most common type of icthyosis—does not usually manifest itself until after six months of age. The pale, flaky scales are
obvious, especially on the outer surfaces of arms and legs; the chest, back,
and face tend to be less affected. Armpit, elbow, and groin creases are also
usually free of scales. Histologically, there is a marked thickening of a
particular part of the skin—the stratum corneum.

Lamellar icthyosis is usually obvious at birth and has led to the term "collodion baby." Large plate-like scales are found all over the body at birth. This condition will have a number of adverse effects when, for example, the nostrils are blocked by thick scales; ears are similarly blocked; or sweat glands are obstructed by the thickened skin. Babies born with this type of icthyosis can be extremely ill if respiration is impeded by thickened scales in the nose. Histologically, there is a very thick stratum corneum. (This type is inherited in an autosomal recessive manner.)

Bullous icthyosis is also obvious at birth, with reddened skin underlying thick warty scales. Blistering of the abnormal skin occurs in the early months of life, but this problem frequently ceases after the age of one year. Again, histologically, there is a very thick stratum corneum with also a thickened epidermis and chronic inflammation in the dermis.

MANAGEMENT IMPLICATIONS

Emollient creams are necessary throughout life and can control satisfactorily the less severe types of icthyosis. Creams to reduce thickened layers (keratolytics) can also be helpful.

Secondary infection in bullous icthyosis will need to be immediately treated and adequately with **antibiotics.** Disinfectant lotions and creams are helpful and discourage secondary bacterial infection.

The effects on **breathing, hearing,** and/or **sweating** will need specialized and urgent treatment in the lamellar type of icthyosis. Such problems will need monitoring and treating throughout life. Many children show signs of failing to thrive with this condition.

THE FUTURE

Regretfully, spontaneous improvement does not occur with any of the icthyoses, and treatment will need to be life-long. Careers must be carefully chosen to avoid further damage to the abnormal skin.

SELF-HELP GROUP

F.I.R.S.T.
Foundation for Ichthyosis and Related Skin Types
P.O. Box 669
Ardmore, PA 19003
610-789-3995 or 800-545-3286
http://www.libertynet.org/icthyos
email: Ichthyosis@aol.com

Johanson–Blizzard Syndrome

ALTERNATIVE NAME

Ectodermal dysplasia-pancreatic insufficiency.

INCIDENCE

Johanson–Blizzard syndrome is rare, but it has been well documented. Both boys and girls can be affected.

HISTORY

This syndrome was classified and documented in the early 1970s by Drs. Johanson and Blizzard of the USA.

CAUSATION

Johanson–Blizzard syndrome is thought to be inherited in an autosomal recessive way. There have been reports of more than one affected child in a family, and consanguinity has also been reported as a possible factor.

At present there are no prenatal tests available. Genetic counseling before further pregnancy is advisable.

CHARACTERISTICS

Unusual facial features are obvious at birth. The baby's nose is small and short from base to tip, and the upper jaw is small. Microcephaly can also, but not inevitably, be present.

Teeth when they erupt are small and widely spaced, and may be absent altogether in some parts of the mouth.

Failure to thrive early on in life is due to **malabsorption of food,** which is caused by a deficiency in the pancreatic enzymes specifically concerned with the breakdown and absorption of food. Glucose tolerance tests and sweat tests (cf. cystic fibrosis) are usually normal. This finding suggests secretions from the pancreas are not completely absent; instead, there is only a variable deficiency.

Learning difficulties can occur, although they do not affect all persons with Johanson–Blizzard syndrome.

Other features that can occur with this syndrome are: sensorineural deafness; under-activity of the thyroid gland, which gives rise to hypothyroidism; general poor muscle tone; possible abnormalities around the anal region (such as an imperforate anus); and a greater susceptibility to respiratory infections.

All these latter features will not necessarily affect each and every affected baby, but they must be remembered as possibilities when caring for children with this syndrome. The three characteristics—unusual facial features, small teeth, and pancreatic insufficiency—must all be present before a diagnosis of Johanson–Blizzard syndrome is made.

MANAGEMENT IMPLICATIONS

The most urgent treatment will be to correct the **food malabsorption** due to the pancreatic insufficiency. Pancreatic enzymes will need to be given orally on a daily basis and a specialized diet must be followed—this latter being adjusted to the child's growing needs as the years pass. Vitamin intake—especially of the fat-soluble ones—also needs to be closely monitored. Even with good dietary control, growth will be slow, and final weight and height will be below average.

Replacement thyroxine, if the thyroid gland is under-active, will also be needed on a daily basis.

In severe cases of **nasal abnormality,** corrective surgery may be needed.

Learning difficulties will need assessment by a multidisciplinary team as the child grows and develops. Depending on the degree and nature of the disability, specialized teaching may need to be arranged.

Respiratory infections, which appear to occur more commonly and frequently than usual, will need adequate treatment.

THE FUTURE

Life expectancy may be reduced if respiratory infections are severe. Lifestyle will depend on the degree and type of learning disability.

SELF-HELP GROUPS

There is no known U.S. organization dedicated to Johanson–Blizzard syndrome, but the following groups may offer assistance:

National Organization for Rare Disorders, Inc. (NORD)
P.O. Box 8923
New Fairfield, CT 06812-8923
203-746-6518 or 800-999-6673
http://www.nord-rdb.com/~orphan
email: orphan@nord-rdb.com

FACES: The National Craniofacial Association
P.O. Box 11082
Chattanooga, TN 37401
423-266-1632
http://www.faces-cranio.org
email: faces@faces-cranio.org

Kartagener Syndrome

ALTERNATIVE NAMES

Immotile cilia syndrome; primary ciliary dyskinesia.

INCIDENCE

There are no exact figures for the number of people affected by this syndrome, but it is thought that as many as 1 child in every 4,000 could be affected. Both boys and girls can suffer from Kartagener syndrome.

HISTORY

In 1933, Dr. Kartagener noticed the relationship between frequent lung and sinus infections and certain specific abnormalities of internal organs, namely, the switching of position of some organs to the opposite side of the body. Abnormally positioned organs could include the heart; this organ, under these circumstances, is situated on the right side of the chest.

In 1970, the basic problem causing the recurrent sinus and chest infections was found to be an abnormality in the cilia in certain parts of the body. (Cilia are the minute hairs to be found primarily in all parts of the respiratory tract, as well as in other parts of the body. Their function is to sweep secretions up and out of the respiratory tract by beating gently backwards and forwards.) In this syndrome, the cilia are comparatively immobile, effectively preventing mucus being removed from the respiratory tract. This static mucus then readily becomes infected, giving rise to the well-known symptoms of upper and lower respiratory tract infections.

The situs invertus (internal organs on the incorrect side of the body) originally noted by Dr. Kartagener has been found to occur in only some sufferers from Kartagener syndrome.

CAUSATION

This condition has recently been found to have an autosomal recessive inheritance. There is no diagnostic prenatal test available as yet.

CHARACTERISTICS

Babies with this syndrome will commonly have some breathing problems at birth, due to difficulties in moving their normal secretions. However, this condition quickly improves with appropriate neonatal care. There are often few indications that the child has any specific condition until the early toddler years, although the young baby often has thick secretions constantly running from his/her nose. He/she may also suffer from a seemingly permanently blocked nose, which can cause problems with feeding.

During the toddler years, the child will suffer from **frequent upper and lower respiratory tract infections.** Many children do, of course, suffer from frequent coughs and colds at this time of their lives. The child with Kartagener syndrome, however, will have an almost perpetually running nose, with thick mucus a constant problem. He/she will also have a constant loose cough. The upper respiratory tract infections will frequently extend down into the lungs, with the risk of resultant pneumonia.

Ear infections associated with these bouts of respiratory infection are common. The thick mucus retained in the middle ear following these infections can lead to a conductive deafness.

Sinusitis is often associated with infections, causing headaches and pain in the cheek regions.

Lack of a sense of **smell** is another common associated problem. In addition to missing out on a good deal of pleasure, the person lacking a normal sense of smell may not be alerted to the potential dangers of, for example, leaking gas or spoiled food.

Bronchiectasis can be the end result of the frequent lung infections. In this condition, the walls of the alveoli of the lungs are destroyed. The condition effectively reduces the oxygen-exchanging capability of the lungs, and it also allows extra excess mucus to accumulate. These lung changes will only occur after a number of years of repeated infection.

Situs invertus is commonly present in children with this syndrome, but it does not inevitably occur. The organs involved can vary; for example, only the heart (dextrocardia—the heart on the right) is involved in some children. Other abdominal organs can also be reversed. Few symptoms need result from these anomalies, but additional heart defects also can occasionally be present.

Symptoms of Kartagener syndrome vary, ranging from severe lung problems to only mild recurring lung infections, and the above anomalies may not be linked together for a number of years. When it is realized that they may be connected, it is possible, by electron microscopy, to test the mobility of the cilia. A sample of cilia can be obtained by a nasal scraping. This test is expensive and requires skilled interpretation.

Infertility in men is one further problem associated with Kartagener syndrome. The tail of the sperm has an almost identical structure to that of the cilia in other parts of the body. For normal fertilization to occur, this tail needs to be active, but in Kartagener syndrome, this activity is much reduced.

MANAGEMENT IMPLICATIONS

Antibiotic treatment, when necessary for severe respiratory tract infections, should be continued for an adequate length of time with maximal doses. Due to the thick secretions found in Kartagener syndrome, penetration by the antibiotics can be difficult.

Physical therapy is valuable for the child who is severely affected and unable to cough up his/her sticky secretions. Postural drainage, two or three times a day, will help to prevent build-up of mucus and reduce infection to a minimum. This treatment is especially important in young children, so that later bronchiectasis can be avoided. By the age of nine to ten years, children can themselves learn techniques to clear their chests effectively.

Physical activities should be encouraged in children with this syndrome, provided that there is no other medical reason, such as a heart defect, for the child to avoid of physical activity. Outdoor games and similar active pursuits are especially valuable.

Hearing should be checked regularly in all children who have associated frequent attacks of otitis media. If a hearing disability occurs during the active time of speech development—between one and three years—there may be delay in acquisition of this skill. Following treatment of the hearing problem, speech therapy may be necessary.

Myringotomy to drain excess fluid from the middle ear may also be necessary. Some authorities advocate the insertion of ventilation tubes to promote drainage of this fluid.

Heart defects, if present, will need appropriate treatment.

THE FUTURE

The future will depend on the severity of the ciliary abnormality. Some people will only be mildly irritated by their frequent nasal and sinus infections. Others will be frequently incapacitated by severe lung infections, and the effects of bronchiectasis. Due to these lung problems, smoking is inadvisable. The effects of the nicotine will inhibit he action of the cilia in the lungs even further.

Lack of a sense of smell, and a mild hearing loss, may pass unnoticed unless specifically tested.

Some men will be infertile due to this syndrome.

Life expectancy is not reduced, unless there are associated heart abnormalities, or the bronchiectasis is very severe.

SELF-HELP GROUPS

There are no known groups in the United States dedicated to Kartagener syndrome, but the following organizations may offer assistance:

National Organization for Rare Disorders, Inc. (NORD)
P.O. Box 8923
New Fairfield, CT 06812-8923
203-746-6518 or 800-999-6673
http://www.nord-rdb.com/~orphan
email: orphan@nord-rdb.com

American Lung Association
1740 Broadway
New York, NY 10019
212-315-8700
http://www.lungusa.org
email: info@lungusa.org

Klinefelter Syndrome

ALTERNATIVE NAME

Chromosome XXY.

INCIDENCE

The incidence of Klinefelter syndrome is surprisingly high. According to chromosomal studies on newborn babies, approximately 1 in every 500 boys have the typical chromosomal pattern associated with this syndrome. In institutions for mentally retarded adults, around one in every 100 men are found to have this chromosomal abnormality.

HISTORY

The typical characteristics of this syndrome were first described by Drs. Klinefelter and Albright in 1942.

CAUSATION

An extra X chromosome is the usual pattern in this syndrome (normal sex chromosomes for males are XY; for females, they are XX). The presence of the extra chromosome is caused by a complex fault in the cell division of one of the parent's sex cells, either the ovum or the sperm, that goes to form the new baby.

There is also a "mosaic" form of Klinefelter syndrome in which only some of the body cells have an XXY chromosome pattern, the remainder having the normal XY count. (There can also be more complex chromosomal abnormalities, the resultant chromosomal pattern being XXXY or even XXXXY, but these abnormalities are unusual.)

Broadly speaking, the severity of the characteristics will depend on the number of cells in the body that have the abnormal chromosome pattern.

CHARACTERISTICS

The signs and symptoms of this condition vary widely from individual to individual. The description below lists all the effects that are a possibility.

All these signs and symptoms will not necessarily be seen in any one individual.

At birth, and during early childhood, there is no obvious evidence of any abnormality, apart from the chance finding of the testes being smaller than is usual. It is at puberty that the following changes become obvious.

The **testes** and **penis** of the boy with Klinefelter syndrome are small. This decreased size of the sex organs persists into adult life, when there is also a marked disturbance of sexual function. Infertility, impotence, and decreased libido all result from this chromosomal abnormality. Blood tests show increased levels of gonadotropins and a decreased level of testosterone.

A feminine type of **breast development** is often obvious in boys with Klinefelter syndrome.

Tall stature is another consistent features of the syndrome. The body proportions are unusual: the legs are disproportionately long when compared with the trunk.

Body hair is usually scanty in boys with Klinefelter syndrome. Normal pubic, axillary, and chest hair fails to appear, and daily shaving is rarely necessary.

Mental abilities are often at the low end of normal. Verbal skills seem to be especially affected in boys with Klinefelter syndrome.

Psychological difficulties, due to the unusual sexual characteristics, are common when adolescence is reached. These difficulties persist into adult life and can merge into serious psychiatric problems.

Diabetes and **thyroid problems** are more common than usual in boys and men with Klinefelter syndrome.

MANAGEMENT IMPLICATIONS

The most serious effect of Klinefelter syndrome is the **psychological trauma** felt by many boys at puberty when secondary sexual characteristics do not develop along normal lines. Testes and penis do not enlarge; pubic and axillary hair does not grow; and breast development is more feminine than most boys would wish. Add to these developmental problems, in many cases, slow mental ability, and the scene is set for much psychological unhappiness. Boys may seek ways to avoid the hurtful teasing to which they are frequently subjected, and secondary behavioral problems often occur. For example, the boy may become the class clown, or he may commit antisocial acts in an endeavor to gain in some way the commendation of his peers.

A **clinical psychologist** can be of great value in helping the boy with Klinefelter syndrome come to terms with his genetic inheritance.

Testosterone therapy should be given from 11 to 12 years on. This treatment will aid the development of more normal sexual characteristics, although it will have no effect on the infertility. Testosterone therapy can help to reduce the psychological problems encountered during adolescence and early adult life.

Schooling: attendance at a mainstream school is usually possible for most boys with Klinefelter syndrome, although some individuals with more restricted intellectual abilities will need special facilities. The increased possibility of diabetes or thyroid imbalance must also be remembered.

THE FUTURE

All boys with Klinefelter syndrome are infertile, and only four men with the mosaic form of the syndrome have been known to father children.

Career choices may well be limited by reduced mental abilities and also by the difficult behavior found in some men and boys with this syndrome.

Life expectancy is thought to be normal.

SELF-HELP GROUP

Klinefelter Syndrome and Associates
P.O. Box 119
Roseville, CA 95678-0119
916-773-2999
http://www.genetic.org/ks/
email: ksinfo@genetic.org

Klippel–Feil Syndrome

ALTERNATIVE NAMES

Klippel–Feil anomaly; congenital brevicollis; Klippel–Feil sequence; Klippel–Feil disorder.

INCIDENCE

The reported incidence of Klippel–Feil syndrome is around 1 in 40,000 live births; girls are affected more often than boys (in an approximate ratio of 60 to 40). It is thought that many more children than this figure would suggest are mildly affected, but the abnormality is of such a mild degree as to pass unnoticed.

A number of different types of the condition have been described, depending on which part of the upper spine is most involved.

CAUSATION

Most cases of this syndrome are thought to arise sporadically, but there are some reports of families in which there are a number of affected individuals. These family histories point to an autosomal dominant or an autosomal recessive inheritance. It is thought that there may be two separate single-gene forms of Klippel–Feil syndrome.

Prenatal scanning can sometimes pick up the spinal abnormalities.

CHARACTERISTICS

The most usual form of Klippel–Feil syndrome is characterized by the fusion of one or more of the cervical or thoracic vertebrae, which creates a **short neck** with folds of skin passing to the shoulders to give a webbed appearance. **Neck movements** are limited, particularly the side-to-side and rotational movements. Flexion and extension movements are often easily performed. (Occasionally, the abnormal fusion of the vertebrae extends to those lower in the spine—the lower thoracic region or even the lumbar region. Under these circumstances, movement in these parts of the spine would also be limited.) This limitation of movement is not painful, as it can be with arthritis, for example.

The importance of this abnormality lies in the complications that can occur when the spinal cord, which is so closely encased in the vertebrae, is injured. Symptoms can range from numbness and tingling in arms and fingers to spasticity or paralysis. These symptoms can arise quite spontaneously, or they can be the result of only a minor fall, stumble, or knock. The vertebrae that are actually fused are not the problem; rather the adjacent ones become excessively mobile in an attempt to mobilize the whole spine, and when these mobile vertebrae move out of position, they can damage the enclosed spinal cord. These symptoms most frequently occur between 10 and 20 years of age, years of maximum activity.

A **low hair-line** at the back of the neck is a classic sign of Klippel–Feil syndrome.

This triad of signs—a short, webbed neck, a low hair-line, and limited neck movements make up the classic picture of Klippel–Feil syndrome.

Other **bony abnormalities,** including scoliosis, extra ribs in the cervical region, and Sprengel shoulder (one shoulder higher than the other) are also sometimes seen.

Other more unusual associated abnormalities can include:

- defects in the **urinary system,** such as horseshoe kidneys;
- **eye** problems, such as lazy eye, nystagmus, or ptosis;
- **cleft palate;**
- **deafness** of either a sensorineural or a conductive type;
- **cardiac abnormalities,** particularly ventricular septal defects.

Each of these associated characteristics affects only a small proportion of persons with Klippel–Feil syndrome, and they certainly would not all occur together in one individual.

MANAGEMENT IMPLICATIONS

The fusion of the cervical vertebrae and the relative instability of the adjacent vertebrae must always be borne in mind when caring for a child with Klippel–Feil syndrome. Contact sports in which the cervical spine, or indeed any part of the spine, could be damaged must be avoided. Interests in more sedentary activities should be encouraged. If damage to the spinal cord does occur, either spontaneously or as the result of injury, urgent surgical stabilization is necessary.

Other **bony abnormalities,** such as scoliosis or Sprengel shoulder, may also need surgical intervention to prevent the deformity from worsening and/or to further improve mobility.

Any **renal abnormality** giving rise to symptoms—perhaps increased liability to urinary infection, for example—must be investigated and remedied where possible.

Deafness must be remembered as a possibility in children with Klippel–Feil syndrome. Hearing should be checked if there is any suspicion that a child is not hearing properly.

Lazy eye should be treated early, if present, to prevent amblyopia occurring.

A **cleft palate,** if present, will also need surgical repair. Subsequent speech therapy may be needed to ensure correct speech.

THE FUTURE

Children with Klippel–Feil syndrome can look forward to a normal life span, provided there are no serious associated kidney problems. Care must be taken at all times to avoid excessive trauma to the neck. For example, adequate head restraints should be fitted to any car in which the child, and later the adult, is traveling.

Careers, too, must be chosen with these potential problems in mind.

SELF-HELP GROUP

Klippel–Feil Syndrome Support Group
311 Bracken Avenue
Pittsburgh, PA 15527
412-884-2969

Landau–Kleffner Syndrome

ALTERNATIVE NAMES

Infantile acquired aphasia; aphasia with convulsive disorder.

INCIDENCE

Landau–Kleffner syndrome is a rare disorder. Children between the ages of 3 and 8 years are commonly affected, with the condition often appearing in the preschool years. Both boys and girls can be affected with the condition; at present, twice as many girls as boys are affected.

HISTORY

Landau–Kleffner syndrome was first described in 1957 by Dr. William Landau and Dr. Frank Kleffner, who identified six children in their practice with the condition. Since that time, a number of other children have been diagnosed.

CAUSATION

The basic cause of Landau–Kleffner syndrome is unknown. It is not thought to be a genetic disorder because family studies have not shown signs of the disease in other family members. One theory of causation, however, considers that this condition is a manifestation of the extreme end of the large group of genetic epilepsies. The other theory suggests that a localized inflammation of the small blood vessels in the brain causes the syndrome. Research is continuing into other possible etiological factors.

CHARACTERISTICS

As one of the alternative names for this syndrome—"infantile acquired aphasia"—implies, the child will initially develop quite normally. Then, either suddenly or over a comparatively brief period of time—and for no apparent reason—the child will have **difficulty in understanding what is said.** Initially, and understandably, this difficulty is often thought to be due to an onset of deafness, but hearing tests show no evidence of hearing loss.

Along with the lack of comprehension of the spoken word will eventually arise an **inability to communicate.** In a young child in whom speech is not yet secure, this aspect of the syndrome can be difficult to differentiate from other possible causes affecting the production of speech—such as an intercurrent infection for example.

Older children who have learned to read and write before the onset of this unusual condition will usually be able to communicate in writing, and other children can make themselves understood by gesture or sign language. It appears that it is only the ability to speak that is affected.

Along with the loss of language, the child will experience **epileptic seizures.** These may begin before the speech problem becomes obvious, or they may occur at much the same time. The type of seizure is very variable and can range from petit mal (or "absences") to generalized seizures or partial seizures affecting only, for example, the face. In the most severely affected children, seizures can become continuous and lead to status epilepticus, which will require urgent medical treatment. It is thought that this severe condition will occur in around 15% of children with Landau–Kleffner syndrome. A further difficulty in diagnosis is that the seizures frequently only occur at night.

Behavioral difficulties, ranging from autistic behavior to excessive and/or unusual behavior patterns, can arise. (Such problems, of course, are very understandable in a child who has suddenly lost the ability to speak.)

INVESTIGATIONS

EEG will show specific changes. Readings should be taken during sleep because it is at this time that most seizures or alterations in brainwave patterns will occur.

MANAGEMENT IMPLICATIONS

Anticonvulsant drugs will be needed to control seizures. It is possible that a number of different drugs will need to be tried before the right drug, or combination of drugs, is found to suit the individual child. Control of the seizures appears to have little effect on the child's subsequent language ability.

Steroids have improved the speech problems in some cases. These powerful drugs will need to be used with caution in young children, and the child must be monitored closely for their side effects.

Help with language and speech skills is important to the ultimate outcome of this condition. Each child's specific needs will require assessment by an experienced speech and language therapist before decisions are made as to the most useful form of treatment. Intensive programs, including specific auditory training and signing and visual sequencing methods, will need to be formalized. Older children who are able to read and write will need emphasis to be put on these skills.

Behavior modification techniques can also be of value if this aspect of Landau–Kleffner syndrome causes particular difficulty.

THE FUTURE

The majority of children outgrow the seizures by the time they are 15 years old At this time, EEG recordings are found to be normal.

The recovery of language is less predictable and can range from a reported few children who have complete language recovery to others who never recover any verbal communication—with all stages in between. Severely affected children often find life in a deaf community where sign language is the norm more comfortable than life among speaking peers.

A normal life span is expected.

SELF-HELP GROUPS

C.A.N.D.L.E.
4414 McCampbell Drive
Montgomery, AL 36106
334-271-3947

Epilepsy Foundation
4351 Garden City Drive
Landover, MD 20785-2267
301-459-3700 or 800-332-1000

Laurence–Moon–Bardet–Biedl Syndrome

ALTERNATIVE NAMES

Current thinking now subdivides this syndrome into two separate entities—Laurence–Moon syndrome and Bardet–Biedl syndrome. As there is much overlap of symptoms between these two syndromes, they will be described together, with references being given where they diverge.

The syndrome can be known as LMBBS.

INCIDENCE

Incidence is variable in different parts of the world. In Newfoundland, the prevalence is considered to be around 1 in 17,500. Among Bedouin populations in Kuwait, LMBBS is seen in the order of 1 in 13,500. In both these cases, consanguinity is thought to have a strong bearing on the incidence.

In Europe, the incidence is much lower. A recent British study estimated the incidence to be as low as 1 in 125,000.

Both sexes are equally affected.

HISTORY

Dr. John Zachariah Laurence, a London ophthalmologist, and his house surgeon, Dr. Robert Moon, first reported on the typical features of the syndrome in the latter part of the 19th century.

In the early 1920s, Dr. George Bardet described some of the clinical features, as did Dr. Arthur Biedl a few years later. They did not refer to the previous work of Laurence and Moon. In 1925, two other doctors looked at both these reports and considered the conditions reported to be the same. Hence, the name Laurence–Moon–Bardet–Biedl syndrome came into being.

As has already been mentioned, it is only recently that the syndrome has been split into two separate entities—namely Laurence–Moon syndrome and Bardet–Biedl syndrome. This distinction has been made because the incidence of the clinical features seen in the two conditions, although they have much in common, do vary both in severity and type.

This situation is confusing, making diagnosis in individual cases difficult.

CAUSATION

The mode of inheritance is autosomal recessive. In 1993 and succeeding years, the gene loci have been reported to be on four different sites on chromosomes 16, 11, 3, and 15. The way in which the faulty genes cause the disease is still to be elucidated, although it is thought that some enzyme defect is the basis of the diverse symptoms seen.

When one child in the family has the syndrome, each future pregnancy runs a 25% risk of having another affected child, so genetic counseling is advisable.

CHARACTERISTICS

There is wide variation in the symptoms seen in these syndromes. Before a diagnosis is secure, four of the following features will need to be present. Other secondary characteristics may also apply to each individual child; these secondary characteristics will determine, to some extent, the classification of the syndrome.

All children who are diagnosed as having either Laurence–Moon syndrome or Bardet–Biedl syndrome will show at least four of the following characteristics:

Visual difficulties in the form of "rod–cone dystrophy," in which there is an abnormality in some of the cells that make up the retina. This condition will initially mean that the child will have difficulty in seeing in the dark; the visual handicap will eventually devolve into complete night blindness. Daytime vision is present, but it is poor in the early years and will slowly deteriorate over the succeeding years. The rate of this progression will vary from individual to individual, but many children will be registered as legally blind by the time they are 15 years of age.

Obesity. This problem arises early on in life, and, in spite of adequate dietary control, it is difficult to treat.

Polydactyly (extra fingers and toes). This condition may take the form of a small skin tag or a fully formed finger or toe, usually on the outer side of the hand or foot. Toes and fingers also tend to be short and stubby.

Sex organs—especially noticeable in boys—are small and underdeveloped. This characteristic is present from birth, but it will become more obvious in boys later in life when there is lack of development of penis and testes.

Learning disability is frequently present, although to a variable degree. Routine developmental checks are advisable early on in life to identify other problems that may be masked originally by the visual impairment.

Kidney abnormalities can be present, leading to renal excretory problems These can vary from a mild reflux problem with frequent attacks of urinary infection to other more serious structural abnormalities, which will require the careful constant monitoring of kidney function together with routine blood pressure measurements.

Other signs and symptoms include **poor coordination** and clumsiness, which—rarely and only in the severely affected child—can lead to ataxia, which can be progressive and lead to spasticity.

Speech difficulties can occur.

Diabetes, usually of the noninsulin dependent type, can be a problem.

MANAGEMENT IMPLICATIONS

Visual difficulties will become more apparent as the child matures. Sight will initially be adequate centrally, but peripheral vision will be limited. Central vision will also eventually become diminished, in spite of efforts to halt the process. Other eye signs, such as lazy eye or nystagmus, may also be present. Electroretinography (ERG) and visually evoked response (VER) are useful tests to determine the degree of visual loss.

It is important that children are prepared for other ways of obtaining information other than sight—such as learning Braille.

The **obesity** can be difficult to manage. A mixture of a dietitian's advice and encouragement to take sufficient exercise—within the constraints of the other disabilities—is probably the best way to treat this problem. It may be necessary to try appetite suppressants if the problem becomes unmanageable by other means.

Extra fingers and toes need to be treated surgically—skin tags can be tied off early in life, while extra digits need surgery within the first few years. It is important that extra fingers and toes are removed as these can be a source of discomfort in, for example, any activity using fine motor skills. Extra toes can also cause problems with fitting of shoes.

Hypogonadism can be stressful for individuals with LMBBS around the time of puberty, and especially so for boys. There is little that can be done to increase the size of the penis or testes. Testosterone has been tried, but with little effect.

Learning difficulties will need ongoing assessment so that help can be given in any areas in which the child lags behind peers. Once school days arrive, the most appropriate school needs to be chosen. Many children with LMBBS manage initially in mainstream school when extra help is available. This help is especially necessary for children with speech difficulties and for those in whom visual deterioration is rapid.

Renal problems will need treatment if, and when, they arise. Treatment will depend on the type and severity of the kidney abnormality. Renal ultrasound will help to determine the extent of any difficulties.

Coordination difficulties and/or clumsiness must be taken into account when assessing the child with LMBBS Difficulties can arise when trying to suggest appropriate exercise for overweight children if poor coordination is also present.

The possible onset of **diabetes** must always be remembered, and regular tests for urinary sugar are advisable.

THE FUTURE

Careers must be geared to the expected gradual loss of vision and also to any learning disability present. Help from organizations for the blind can be helpful.

Males are likely to be infertile, although it is possible that they can father children. Women, if there are no structural abnormalities in the reproductive tract, can give birth to healthy children.

SELF-HELP GROUPS

Laurence–Moon–Bardet–Biedl Syndrome
c/o The Foundation Fighting Blindness
Executive Plaza 1
11350 McCormick Road, Suite 800
Hunt Valley, MD 21031
410-785-1414
http://www.blindness.org
email: mmarzullo@blindness.org

Lennox–Gastaut Syndrome

ALTERNATIVE NAME

"Malignant epilepsy."

INCIDENCE

As the alternative name to this syndrome implies, Lennox–Gastaut syndrome is a severe form of childhood epilepsy. The actual incidence of the condition is not known, but it is thought that around 10% of children with epilepsy have this syndrome, and that up to 50% of children who have epileptic seizures that are difficult to treat have this syndrome.

Although certain criteria must be met before this particular syndrome can be recognized (see below), many authorities consider that this syndrome should be classed under the general heading of epilepsy. It is, however, useful to consider this syndrome as a specific entity when discussing prognosis and treatment.

Boys and girls are equally affected. The features of this syndrome become apparent between the ages of 3 and 10 years—most usually when a child is 4 to 5 years old.

There is no prenatal diagnosis possible.

CAUSATION

There are a number of events that may possibly be involved in the etiology of this syndrome:

- Lennox–Gastaut syndrome can occur in children with existing brain damage.
- In up to one-quarter of cases, the child had infantile spasms ("salaam attacks") in earlier childhood (see West syndrome). It is thought possible that Lennox–Gastaut syndrome is a later manifestation of this latter syndrome.
- The child showing the typical epileptic pattern of Lennox–Gastaut syndrome may also have other neurological conditions, such as a brain tumor, a previous severe head injury, a subdural hematoma, or a congenital condition such as tuberous sclerosis.

- It is thought possible that genetic factors could account for a small number of cases—around 3%.

CHARACTERISTICS

There are four features that lead to a diagnosis of Lennox–Gastaut syndrome:

- **frequent seizures** of types varying from recurrent "absences" through convulsive fits to non-convulsive "status epilepticus";
- the **electroencephalogram** shows a pattern typical of the condition;
- the **seizures are especially difficult to control** and are resistant to many of the known anticonvulsant drugs;
- most children with this syndrome will be **mentally retarded.**

Because the seizures occur in so many random different ways, it can be difficult to diagnose this syndrome. Children can suffer from the most widely known type of seizure (where a fall to the ground is followed by twitching movements). This type of seizure can occur during sleep, which can add to the diagnostic problems. Other children who show the typical EEG pattern of Lennox–Gastaut syndrome can have very frequent attacks (sometimes so frequent as to be almost continuous) of "absences" with head nodding, eye blinking, a lack of facial expression, and drooling. Yet others suffer from "drop" attacks, where there is a sudden unexpected fall to the ground. This latter type of seizure can occur with, or without, twitching movements.

In addition to these frequent seizures, the child can develop **behavioral problems.** These can include many autistic features as well as many bizarre mannerisms. These problems can be especially difficult to handle if they are first manifested when the child is playing with others or in an early school situation before a definitive diagnosis has been made.

Intelligence will gradually deteriorate with the continuation of the seizures. The cause of this unhappy development is not clear. It may be that the continual seizures damage brain function, or it may be that both the seizures and the mental retardation have a common underlying pathological cause.

INVESTIGATIONS

The electroencephalogram will show the typical pattern associated with this syndrome.

MANAGEMENT IMPLICATIONS

First and foremost, all efforts must be made to control seizures with **anticonvulsant drugs.** As mentioned before, achieving control can be extremely difficult and may never be wholly successful. It is vital that the child's medication is kept under regular review. Steroids have been tried to control the seizures, but they have not been entirely successful.

For the child with frequent "drop" attacks, a well-fitting **protective helmet** is necessary to prevent head injuries.

A **ketogenic diet** has been tried for some children with intractable epilepsy, with varying degrees of success. This diet is high in fats and triglycerides, and it must only be given under a dietitian's and pediatrician's control. (Trials of this diet began when it was noticed that the seizures tended to improve when the child had a febrile illness. Following this observation, a diet that mimicked the physiological conditions seen in a febrile illness was tried.)

Operative procedures on the brain for children with repeated "drop" attacks are currently being evaluated.

Schooling will need to be very specialized to cope with both the frequent seizures and the mental retardation. It is also important to realize that the child's physical state, and hence abilities, can vary markedly from day to day. Close liaison between health and education authorities is vital.

Ideally, arrangements should be made so the rest of the family can occasionally go on vacation free from the responsibility of caring full-time for a handicapped member.

THE FUTURE

Children with Lennox–Gastaut syndrome will need care throughout their lives. Given the difficulties experienced in controlling the seizures and the probable deterioration in intellectual function, an independent life will be impossible.

SELF-HELP GROUPS

Lennox–Gastaut Syndrome Group
6443 Riggs Place
Los Angeles, CA 90045
310-670-8279
email: ANDYDOW@aol.com

Epilepsy Foundation of America
4351 Garden City Drive
Landover, MD 20785
301-459-3700
http://www.efa.org
email: webmaster@efa.org

LEOPARD Syndrome

ALTERNATIVE NAMES

Multiple lentigines syndrome; cardio-cutaneous syndrome.

INCIDENCE

LEOPARD syndrome is a rare condition, the exact incidence of which is not known, but 70 cases have been described in the literature. Both boys and girls can be affected. This syndrome is regarded as an association of abnormalities specifically affecting different parts of the body; LEOPARD is an acronym for *l*entigines (small dark-brown spots); *o*cular features; *p*ulmonary stenosis; *a*bnormalities of genitalia; growth *r*etardation; and *d*eafness.

The name also refers to the vast number of small dark-brown spots seen all over the body, which are reminiscent of the markings of a leopard.

HISTORY

This syndrome was first described in the late 1960s.

CAUSATION

LEOPARD syndrome is inherited as an autosomal dominant characteristic. The degree of expression varies from individual to individual, some family members being more affected than other members. Less severely affected parents can have more severely affected children and vice versa (cf. neurofibromatosis).

CHARACTERISTICS

Lentigines, small, dark-brown spots, are found all over the face and body of the sufferer from LEOPARD syndrome. These spots can be present at birth, or they can appear gradually over the first three or four years of life. By five years of age, these marks are abundant almost everywhere, except on the mucous membranes inside the mouth and eyelids. The marks also appear in less profusion below the knees. Unlike freckles, the spots do not increase in number when the child is out in the sun. They are also darker in color than freckles, and they are always small in size, never being more than 5 millimeters in diameter. The spots are the chief characteristic of LEOPARD syndrome. The other characteristics arise in varying degrees and severity in each individual.

Eyes are widely set apart. Aside from this characteristic, there is no other specific abnormality associated with the eyes, although lazy eye may occasionally be present.

Pulmonary stenosis is often only mild and consists of a narrowing of the pulmonary artery as it arises from the heart. Around 50% of children with LEOPARD syndrome have this abnormality. Even if it is present, this narrowing rarely causes problems. Other conductive conditions in the heart may be seen on EKG tracings, but these problems rarely arise.

Abnormalities in the sex organs include hypospadias, in which the opening of the urethra onto the penis is in an abnormal position, situated not at the tip of the penis but lower down on the shaft of that organ.

Growth retardation is often seen in children with LEOPARD syndrome. The retardation is not excessive, but most children will only reach the 25th percentile on the standard growth charts by the time they are 18 years old.

Deafness affects around one-quarter of children with this syndrome. The hearing disability is sensorineural in type, and it can cause speech delay if it is not noted early.

MANAGEMENT IMPLICATIONS

Nothing can be done about the skin lesions typical of this syndrome. Teasing may occur at school, particularly if the name of the syndrome is known! During the summer months, many other children have a multitude of freckles on their bodies, and at this time of the year, the child with LEOPARD syndrome may be less embarrassed by his/her skin markings.

Lazy eye, if present, should be treated either orthoptically or surgically. Correction should be done early to avoid amblyopia, where vision can be much reduced in one eye. (A lazy eye will cause some degree of double vision. To compensate for this problem, the brain will block off one image, leaving the child with only one visual image. Unless the lazy eye is corrected within a comparatively short time, vision in one eye will disappear altogether through disuse.)

Heart defects will rarely cause any problem. They are often only found later in life, when they are considered an unusual finding, unless, of course, the association with the skin markings is noted.

Hypospadias will need assessment as to its degree and the effect it is having on urine flow. Surgical correction may be needed if the defect is severe. If surgery is necessary, it is wise to perform the operation before the boy starts school, because an unusual flow of urine can cause a small boy much distress.

Deafness will need to be diagnosed and assessed early in the child's life. Speech therapy may be needed during the critical years of speech development (around one to three years of age). Deafness during this important time can easily lead to secondary problems with the acquisition of clear speech.

THE FUTURE

The child with LEOPARD syndrome should experience few difficulties due to his/her genetic inheritance. Deafness may be a factor to be considered in the choice of a career, but apart from this potential problem, a normal life, and life span, can be expected.

SELF-HELP GROUP

There is no known organization in the United States dedicated to LEOPARD syndrome, but the following institution may provide assistance:

National Organization for Rare Disorders, Inc. (NORD)
P.O. Box 8923
New Fairfield, CT 06812-8923
203-746-6518 or 800-999-6673
http://www.nord-rdb.com/~orphan
email: orphan@nord-rdb.com

Lowe Syndrome

ALTERNATIVE NAME

Oculo-cerebro-renal syndrome.

INCIDENCE

Lowe syndrome is a rare syndrome, the exact incidence of which is not known. The basic cause of the condition is thought to be some metabolic disorder. The exact nature of this problem is not clear at present, but research into various areas are proceeding in a number of centers.

Due to the mode of inheritance, only boys are affected.

CAUSATION

Lowe syndrome is inherited as an X-linked recessive disorder. Women who are carriers for the condition occasionally have changes in the lenses of their eyes. These changes rarely cause problems, but they can be an indicator that the family has Lowe syndrome in its genetic inheritance. A family history of present members and ancestors known to have similar characteristics is the best way of estimating the risk to a future pregnancy. There is no prenatal diagnostic test available at present, although the causative gene has now been mapped.

CHARACTERISTICS

As the alternative name suggests, Lowe syndrome affects the eyes, brain, and kidneys of babies with this condition.

Cataracts in both eyes are present at birth in all baby boys with the full expression of Lowe syndrome. The affected lenses are also often small in size.

Glaucoma, in which the tension inside the eyeball is high, is common. It has been suggested that the basic cause for this disease is the small size of the lens, which may effectively block the drainage passages of the eyes.

Lazy eye is similarly common in babies affected by Lowe syndrome.

Nystagmus, a flickering movement (usually horizontal) of the eyes, can be present.

As the baby matures, the eyes do not grow in proportion to the rest of the face, and as a result, the eyes have a sunken appearance later in childhood.

All these potential problems mean that most Lowe children will be blind, or, at best, only partially sighted.

Renal problems: at birth, and for a few weeks afterward, kidney function appears to be normal, but after this time, the tubules in the kidneys fail to function adequately. This failure causes wide-ranging chemical abnormalities due to defective excretion of these substances. The renal problems lead to a number of additional effects, including retarded growth, hypotonic muscles, and a generalized acidosis. The abnormalities in the kidneys become progressively worse as the child matures. Renal failure is frequently seen in mid-childhood.

Mental abilities can vary markedly among boys with Lowe syndrome. A boy may have completely normal mental abilities; he may be very mildly retarded; or he may have a severe mental handicap. Routine developmental testing will bring to light the areas in which help is needed.

MANAGEMENT IMPLICATIONS

Eyes: full assessment by an ophthalmologist is necessary to determine the full extent of the visual handicap. Glaucoma, cataracts, and lazy eye will need to be treated appropriately to ensure that as much vision as possible is saved. Magnification and good lighting will allow the boy to use what vision he has to the best advantage. Regular testing of vision should continue for as long as there is any measurable vision.

Renal problems must also receive skilled care. Correction of acidosis, and the hypophosphatemia that is also a common feature, will increase the quality of life for the child—and his parents. Renal failure must be treated appropriately if and when it arises. Early recognition of renal failure, and subsequent active treatment, can increase life span.

Mental abilities must be checked routinely. All skills, such as walking, speaking, and self-help skills, should be charted. In this way, progress (or the lack of it) can be measured over the years. Regrettably, many of the boys with Lowe syndrome are found to be severely mentally retarded fairly early on in childhood. (However, this condition is by no means invariable, as some boys are able to work and play alongside their peers in spite of their poor vision.) If mental handicap is found to be present, suitable schooling will have to be arranged for the child, either in a special school or in an institution with appropriate facilities.

Behavioral problems can also occur. Frustration, along with a degree of mental handicap, is the most likely cause of this difficult behavior. The help of a clinical psychologist can be valuable under these circumstances.

THE FUTURE

The future is not good for the boy with Lowe syndrome. Many boys die before their tenth birthday, usually from renal failure. Some boys reach adolescence and adulthood. Due to poor vision and possible mental retardation, only very few boys pursue an independent life.

SELF-HELP GROUP

Lowe Syndrome Association
222 Lincoln Street
West Lafayette, IN 47906
http://www.medhelp.org/lowesyndrome
email: lsa@medhelp.org

Marfan Syndrome

ALTERNATIVE NAMES

Arachnodactyly; marfanoid hypermobility syndrome.

INCIDENCE

Marfan syndrome is comparatively common, the condition occurring in at least 1 in every 10,000 persons. Both sexes are equally affected.

HISTORY

Several of the signs of Marfan syndrome are not exclusive to the condition; they are also found among the general population. Therefore, it has been determined that at least three of the specific signs or symptoms associated with the syndrome should be present to accurately and correctly diagnose a person with the condition. If a first-degree relative—i.e. mother, father, brother, or sister—also has Marfan syndrome, only two of the characteristic features are required to make a positive diagnosis.

CAUSATION

Marfan syndrome is inherited as an autosomal dominant, but some cases arise sporadically as new mutations. Even if the abnormal gene is present, all the typical characteristics may not be seen in any one individual. For example, only the tall stature may occur, without the other specific signs.

Recent theories suggest that a particular protein is one of the affected substances producing some of the clinical signs. Similar features to those seen in Marfan syndrome can occur in another disorder, homocystinuria. Amino acid assay of the urine is needed to distinguish between the two disorders.

CHARACTERISTICS

Skeletal system

All children with Marfan syndrome are **tall,** towering over their classmates from an early age. Long, slender limbs, which look out of proportion to normal sized trunks, explain this increased height (cf. achondroplasia).

Vertebral column abnormalities: scoliosis (a sideways bend) can affect the spine in the thoracic region. Kyphosis can also occur in this region of the back, giving rise to the appearance of rounded shoulders.

Fingers and toes are also particularly long and slender—often giving rise to the name of "spider fingers."

Joints are either very mobile or, alternatively, stiff and contracted. The former characteristic is the more common, and it is especially noticeable in the wrists, elbows, and fingers. Dislocation of joints can occur more readily than normal, due to the laxity of the joint capsule and the comparative weakness of the muscles surrounding the joint.

Chest: there are frequently deformities of varying types and degrees in this region of the body.

A **high, arched palate** is a consistent feature.

Eyes

In a high proportion of children with Marfan syndrome, the lenses of the eyes are dislocated, giving rise to poor vision. In addition to that characteristic, myopia (near-sightedness) is common. Detachment of the retina occurs more frequently than in the general population. Lazy eye and/or nystagmus can also occur, but neither is an invariable characteristic.

Cardiovascular system

The upper part of the **aorta,** the large artery passing oxygenated blood from the heart to the rest of the body, is often dilated. This condition can lead to the development of an aneurysm (a "blowing out" of the blood vessel) in later life.

The **valves** of the heart can also be affected, the mitral or aortic valves being the ones most commonly affected. The valves are lax, and they can prolapse, which causes problems of inadequate blood-flow through the heart.

These cardiac defects are all part of the connective tissue disorder.

Mental abilities

Children with Marfan syndrome have normal intelligence. It has been reported that attention span can be limited and that verbal performance, on testing, can lag behind comprehension. These findings do not apply to all children with Marfan syndrome, but there is strong evidence that such mental problems do affect these children more frequently than they affect children in the general population. Therefore, it is important that regular checks on school performance are made.

Other features

Subcutaneous tissue can be reduced, leading to excessive slimness, which adds to the child's long, lean appearance.

Muscles can be weak, so that children with the syndrome are not natural athletes.

MANAGEMENT IMPLICATIONS

Skeletal system

Scoliosis should be noted early before the deformity becomes marked. Scoliosis, if left untreated, can progress to a severe chest deformity with subsequent cardiac and respiratory problems. Therefore, early bracing or operative procedures should be done to reduce the possibility of further problems. Any bracing procedures must, however, be done very carefully, as respiratory problems can result. In girls, early puberty has been induced by the giving of appropriate hormones. This treatment reduces final height, and it can also prevent the worsening of the scoliosis during the period of rapid growth of puberty.

Joint contractures occur in a minority of children. Physical therapy, if given early and consistently, can do much to maintain mobility, which can be at risk due to the joint problems.

Eyes

Early examination of visual acuity is vital, so that corrective lenses can be given to counteract the myopia that is so common.

Lazy eye, if present, will need to be orthoptically or surgically corrected to avoid amblyopia. This treatment is important, as other eye abnormalities already compromise visual acuity in children with Marfan syndrome. Dislocated lenses, which—of course—also reduce vision, should be left in position. In the past, lenses were removed surgically, but it has subsequently been found that this procedure predisposes the person to retinal detachment.

Cardiovascular system

Beta-blocker drugs, given on a long-term basis, have been found to reduce the rate of dilatation of the aorta. Operative procedures may be necessary to replace the dilated aorta at a later date. Some authorities recommend repair of the dilated aorta when the size of this blood vessel has reached 6 centimeters, even if symptoms are not present. Surgery may also be necessary on the abnormal valves in the heart. Endocarditis, an infection of the inner layer of cardiac muscle, is a possible complication. Because of this possibility, antibiotics should be given prophylactically before minor operative procedures, such as dental extractions.

Due to the cardiac, visual, and skeletal problems associated with Marfan syndrome, certain restrictions should be put on affected children's physical activities. For example, contact sports must be avoided due to the possibility of damage to the eyes, and sports that require the body to be pushed to its physical limits, such as marathon running and weightlifting, must be avoided. The heart, under these circumstances, has a heavy load to bear, and with the possible abnormalities to be found in Marfan syndrome, great physical exertion can lead to cardiac failure. Weak muscles and skeletal problems will also, in many cases, exclude many of the more strenuous physical activities.

Mental abilities

Children with Marfan syndrome will be able to manage intellectually in mainstream schooling. Visual problems, however, may be extreme enough that a child will need special schooling.

The possibility of a specific attention deficit must also be remembered; schools should be prepared to take appropriate action to remedy the problem.

THE FUTURE

Children with Marfan syndrome may have a reduced life expectancy due to cardiac problems. The usual life span is 40 to 50 years. Complications arising from aortic abnormalities account for 90% of early deaths. As long as sensible precautions are taken not to overload the cardiovascular system, many individuals can live normal life within the limits of reduced vision. Genetic counseling before a pregnancy is embarked upon is advisable.

SELF-HELP GROUP

National Marfan Foundation
382 Main Street
Port Washington, NY 11050
516-883-8712
http://www.marfan.org
email: staff@marfan.org

Moebius Syndrome

ALTERNATIVE NAMES

Congenital facial diplegia; Moebius sequence.

INCIDENCE

Moebius syndrome is rare, but it nevertheless has important implications for the care of newborn babies. Boys and girls are equally liable to be affected.

A link between Moebius syndrome and two other similar syndromes, the fascinatingly named "Charlie M" syndrome and "Poland" syndrome, has been hypothesized. These two latter syndromes have abnormalities in face, arms, fingers, and chest muscles, as well as facial problems. It has been suggested that a failure of development of specific blood vessels at a critical stage of prenatal life is the basic cause of these abnormalities. Both Charlie M and Poland syndromes are incredibly rare.

CAUSATION

Theories about causation are controversial. Most cases are thought to be sporadic and due to a new mutation, but an autosomal dominant inheritance is also thought to be possible. One family, having the syndrome in three successive generations, had chromosomal abnormalities, but such abnormalities have not been reported again. Yet another suggestion as to the etiology of this syndrome is illness, drug abuse, or an accident affecting the mother during the first three months of pregnancy.

There is no prenatal test available. Moebius syndrome can be recognized at birth by the lack of facial movement.

CHARACTERISTICS

The main effects of Moebius syndrome are found in the **face.** The baby is born with almost complete lack of movement in his/her face, usually on both sides. Little facial expression is ever seen, and the baby's eyes and mouth remain open for most of the time. Occasionally, only the upper part of the face (both sides) is affected. The facial muscles are supplied by specific cranial nerves, arising straight from the brain stem, and studies have been done in relation to these nerves. In a few well-studied cases, the nuclei (the "powerhouse" of the nerve) have been small and underdeveloped.

In addition to weakness of the facial muscles, there is frequently also weakness in muscles of the palate and tongue. All these muscles are intimately connected with sucking and swallowing, and their weakness makes feeding difficult in the newborn baby. Tube feeding may occasionally be necessary to ensure that he/she obtains sufficient nutrition for growth.

Aspiration into the lungs of milk, saliva, or mucus, is a real threat to these young babies. If aspiration occurs, bronchopneumonia can be the result.

As the baby matures, many of these problems improve, although solid food can become lodged in the cheeks of the older child, given the continuing difficulty that child will have with her/his facial muscles.

Eyes must be watched carefully for scratching and possible ulceration of the cornea, which can occur because the baby is unable to close his/her eyes fully. Minute particles of dust in the atmosphere can remain on the delicate tissue of the cornea if they are not washed away by normal blinking.

Speech: difficulties can be experienced in the proper articulation of words because the child's weak facial muscles make it difficult for him/her to move lips and tongue together to shape and form sounds.

Some babies with Moebius syndrome may have abnormalities of the **fingers,** which can be either small and shortened or long and slim.

Chest muscles can also be affected in this syndrome; in some cases, they are absent altogether.

Clubfoot is a finding in 35% of babies with Moebius syndrome.

These three latter aspects overlap with those seen in Poland syndrome.

MANAGEMENT IMPLICATIONS

Most of the acute problems are encountered during the early months of life, **feeding** in particular being a problem. Tube feeding may initially be necessary to prevent aspiration of milk and to avoid exhaustion in the young baby. With weak facial muscles, she or he will have to work twice as hard to gain the same amount of milk as that consumed by more robust babies.

Facial muscles will never be normal, but the baby and older child will eventually learn to cope adequately with swallowing, although sucking may be a continuing problem. Food lodged in cheeks can cause choking in the toddler whose feeding patterns are not fully established.

Therefore, throughout childhood, careful watch must be kept at meal times on children with Moebius syndrome.

Any aspiration problems with the potential to lead to **aspiration pneumonia** must be recognized early and treated energetically.

Early recognition, and treatment, of **corneal abrasions** is vital to prevent corneal scarring. Any redness, excessive watering, or obvious discomfort in the baby's eyes should receive immediate attention.

Speech therapy is of great importance to ensure that the child with Moebius syndrome develops understandable speech. Therapy should be started early, from around 18 months of age. Such an early start will ensure that the child's uncoordinated attempts to pronounce words are reduced to a minimum, and parents will be able to obtain valuable advice on how best they can help their child in this vital skill.

THE FUTURE

Moebius syndrome will not exclude the child and young adult from many activities. However, lack of facial expression and possible difficulties with articulation will obviously make for problems with a career or leisure activity that calls for appearing before the public.

Once the early years are successfully passed, life, and life span, can be practically normal for individuals with Moebius syndrome.

Genetic counseling should be offered to affected families.

SELF-HELP GROUPS

Moebius Syndrome Support Group
38883 Foxholm Drive
Palmade, CA 93551
805-267-2570
http://www.ciacess.com/moebius
email: vmccarrell@mid-mo.com

Moebius Syndrome Foundation
P.O. Box 993
Larchmont, NY 10538
914-834-6008
http://www.ciacess.com/moebius
email: richard_campbell@rcw.org

Morquio Syndrome

ALTERNATIVE NAMES

Mucopolysaccharidosis 4; Brailsford syndrome.

INCIDENCE

Morquio syndrome is one of the mucopolysaccharide abnormalities. The mucopolysaccharides are complex sugars that require a variety of enzymes for their correct metabolism. Each of the diseases in the group known as the mucopolysaccharidoses has a specific enzyme defect. These defects have far-reaching consequences, affecting many organs and tissues of the body. The main problem is the accumulation of mucopolysaccharides in various organs, which gives rise to specific symptoms.

About 1 in 100,000 live births exhibits Morquio syndrome, and both sexes are equally affected.

There appear to be two subtypes of Morquio syndrome: one is milder than the other, but they have similar signs and symptoms.

HISTORY

Morquio initially described a family in which both the parents and the grandparents of the affected child were closely related. This description gave a clue to the genetic basis of the disease. With the advance of biochemical and genetic knowledge, Morquio syndrome has been identified as one of the mucopolysaccharide diseases. (See also Hunter, Hurler, and Sanfilippo syndromes.)

CAUSATION

Morquio syndrome is inherited as an autosomal recessive. The complex sugar involved in this particular mucopolysaccharide disease is keratin sulfate. Excessive amounts of this substance are excreted in the urine of many children affected by Morquio syndrome, but this substance is not found to be present in some children. However, deficiency of the enzyme involved in the metabolism of keratin sulfate can be found by laboratory tests in all cases.

Prenatal diagnosis can be made by chorionic villus sampling or by amniocentesis.

CHARACTERISTICS

Prenatal growth and development proceed normally, and this pattern continues throughout the early months of life. By around 18 months of age, however, the following characteristics begin to appear.

Growth retardation: weight and height development slow down from 18 months or so onwards. By the time the child is five years old, no further growth occurs, and final height rarely reaches more than 32 inches (80 centimeters).

Skeletal changes: the spine and chest can become severely deformed, with marked kyphosis and scoliosis (i.e., the spine is twisted both forwards and sideways). The rib cage is short and broad, and the ribs have a flared appearance at the base. The breast bone is very protruding, giving rise to a pigeon-chested appearance. The neck is shortened, due to failure of proper development of the upper vertebrae. Lack of development of this part of the spine can lead to compression of the spinal cord later in life, giving neurological signs and symptoms in the arms and legs at that time.

Limbs: the arms are relatively long, and all joints are lax, the wrists and fingers being particularly affected. Legs are short, due to the general lack of growth, and knock-knees and flat feet are common.

Teeth, both the first and second set, have abnormal enamel. Due to the lack of protective enamel, infection can be rampant, and tooth decay is a painful, problem.

Deafness is common in children with Morquio syndrome, occurring as a direct result of the accumulation of the specific complex sugar involved in the disease.

Cardiac defects are to found in some children. The most usual problem is failure of development of the aorta.

Eyes: clouding of the cornea, a common occurrence in all the mucopolysaccharide diseases, is frequently seen in children with Morquio syndrome.

The **intelligence** of children with this syndrome develops normally, and so they are able to benefit from normal teaching, within the constraints of their physical capabilities.

Secondary sexual characteristics develop normally.

MANAGEMENT IMPLICATIONS

Spinal problems: the abnormalities in the upper cervical vertebrae frequently give rise to compression of the spinal cord. The compression is due both to the abnormalities in the vertebrae themselves and to the laxity of the ligaments in this part of the body, similar to the lax ligaments around other joints. Weakness in the legs, together with tingling sensations, results from this compression, and without adequate treatment, paralysis can occur. Spinal fusion of the affected vertebrae can prevent, or cure, this problem. Persons caring for children with Morquio syndrome should be aware that this complication can occur and be alerted to the possibility by complaints of increasing weakness in the legs and/or increased difficulty in walking. Physical therapy can be helpful in strengthening leg and arm muscles so that movement is easier. Therapy will also reduce strain on joints with their weak ligaments.

Short stature will create problems with school and work equipment. Specially adapted chairs and tables will help the child with Morquio syndrome as he/she reaches secondary school age. Stairs and long corridors that need to be traversed during the course of a school day can also pose problems. These factors must all be borne in mind when helping the child obtain full benefit from the education system.

Clothing can also be difficult due to the unusual body shape. If at all possible, handmade clothes are most suitable; making well-fitting clothing can be an interesting hobby for children—and adults—with the condition.

Work prospects will depend on finding suitable employment for people of such short stature; other problems such as deafness and possible poor vision may also affect career choices.

Hearing must be assessed regularly. Any loss can be helped by the fitting of hearing aids.

Tooth decay must be treated adequately by regular dental care and the fitting of crowns or dentures where necessary.

THE FUTURE

Life expectancy for the child with Morquio syndrome is reduced by cardiac and neurological complications. For children with the most severe form of the syndrome, these problems frequently lead to death at an early age, usually in the twenties. Persons with the milder type of Morquio syndrome have a longer life expectancy.

SELF-HELP GROUP

National MPS Society, Inc.
102 Aspen Drive
Downington, PA 19335
610-942-0100
http://mpssociety.org
email: presmps@aol.com

Nephrotic Syndrome

ALTERNATIVE NAME

Finnish type nephrosis (primary category only).

INCIDENCE

There are two broad categories of nephrotic syndrome—primary and secondary. The primary type includes nephrosis arising as a congenital abnormality, which was mainly described in Finland (hence the other name of Finnish type nephrosis) The exact incidence of this type is not documented, but both sexes are known to be affected, with perhaps a slight preponderance of boys. Other primary types arise with no known predisposing cause.

Secondary types of nephrotic syndrome can be caused by a variety of infections, such as toxoplasmosis, cytomegalovirus, and syphilis, as well as mercury toxicity and a wide range of other conditions, such as Henoch–Schonlein purpura and other connective tissue disorders.

The overall incidence of nephrotic syndrome differs in various parts of the world, but it is thought to affect around 3 to 4 children in every 100,000 in Caucasian populations. In 1985, a higher incidence was reported among the Asian population in Britain—around 12 to 16 children per 100,000 were suffering from the disease. No account was given for these higher numbers. Many cases in West Africa arise as a result of a particular form of malaria.

CAUSATION

The congenital type of nephrotic syndrome is probably inherited as an autosomal recessive disorder.

As already discussed, there is an enormously wide variety of causes for secondary nephrosis. Some cases also arise completely out of the blue, apparently without any predisposing condition being involved.

The basic pathological changes, giving rise to the typical characteristics of the disease, occur in the kidneys.

CHARACTERISTICS

Whatever the cause of the nephrosis, the same features, due to the **pathological changes in the kidneys,** are always similar.

Signs and symptoms of other underlying conditions—infectious, toxic, or auto-immune, will also be seen in each individual child suffering from the disease.

Swelling, in many parts of the body, is often the very first noticeable feature. Frequently, swelling is especially evident around the child's eyes, causing them to appear as mere slits. Initially, this condition is often attributed to an allergic disorder, but as swelling appears in other parts of the body, the true diagnosis becomes evident.

Fluid can be retained in the lungs and abdomen giving rise to **breathlessness** and/or **abdominal pain.**

The child will be **lethargic** with a **poor appetite,** and may also have bouts of mild **diarrhea.**

Urine output becomes diminished, and the urine that is produced contains much protein.

There is frequently a history of an **upper respiratory tract infection** before these symptoms appear, lending credence to the hypothesis that infection in some way plays a part. (Nephrotic syndrome is characterized by relapses of the disease over the years, and a head cold often seems to be the precipitating factor in the onset of one of these relapses.)

The usual age group of children to be affected is between the ages of 2 and 10 years, with the exception of the congenital type of nephrosis, in which signs of the disease can appear before the age of 3 months.

INVESTIGATIONS

Specialized tests on the **urine** will make the diagnosis clear. **Blood tests** will also be necessary to determine any underlying causes for the onset of the symptoms. Similarly, **throat swabs** can give clues as to possible infectious causes. **Renal biopsy** is sometimes necessary in children where the diagnosis is unclear.

COMPLICATIONS

Extra infection can be a worrying complication of nephrotic syndrome. A certain type of streptococcus bacteria is the most common infecting organism. Peritonitis (infection in the abdominal cavity) is probably one of the most usual—and difficult to diagnose—infections. Diagnosis of the infection can be especially difficult if the child is receiving steroids as part of the treatment for the initial disease, as signs and symptoms of infection are frequently altered by these powerful drugs.

Thrombosis (abnormal clotting) in either veins or arteries is an increased risk for children with nephrotic syndrome, due to the high levels of fibrinogen and other clotting factors seen in this condition. Signs and symptoms will depend on which part of the body is affected.

MANAGEMENT IMPLICATIONS

As mentioned before, a person with nephrotic syndrome will have remissions and relapses. The long, drawn-out sequence of events in this chronic disease can be very frustrating and wearing for both parents and child.

During the initial attack, parents will need full explanation of:

- the likely course of the disease;
- the effects of treatment;
- danger signs to watch for in the everyday life of their child.

In view of the importance of this educational process, it is preferable that the child should initially be in the hospital. It is also easier to stabilize the child on a diet and drug regime on an in-patient basis.

Diet: It is important that an adequate diet is taken to ensure proper growth. The child with nephrotic syndrome will probably have a poor appetite due to the unpleasant features of the disease, so tempting dishes are important. Foods high in salt, including potato chips and many other snack foods, must be avoided. (Dietary restrictions will not prove popular, but they must be observed.) A dietitian's help is of great value in the preparation of suitable and attractive meals.

Careful control of **fluid intake** also plays an important part in the control of the disease. The amount of fluid taken each day must be worked out to cause maximum effect without rendering the child dehydrated. Again, parents must be made aware of the need for these restrictions when the child returns home. Diuretics (fluid removing drugs) may occasionally be needed, but they must be used with caution.

Steroids, given orally, are the first-line drugs to be used in this condition. The dosage given must be carefully controlled and monitored. In most children, the course of the disease will be altered by these powerful drugs. Repeated urine tests, along with the clinical condition of the child, will determine the efficacy of this drug.

Steroids are drugs that benefit many conditions, but they also have side effects, some of which are dangerous. Parents should be warned that:

- their child will have an increased appetite, so they will have to be especially careful regarding snack foods;

- energy levels will increase; parents will notice a great change from the lethargic child they knew before treatment was started;
- it is dangerous to stop taking steroids abruptly. It is important to warn doctors, in cases of accident, that the child needs these drugs;
- they should report to their doctor any close contact the child has had with measles or chickenpox. These two childhood illnesses will be very severe—and can prove to be fatal—for people taking steroids unless preventative action is taken. Under these circumstances, passive immunization with immunoglobulin and/or specific antiviral therapy will be needed. Teaching staff at the child's school will also need to be aware of the dangers to the child of contact with these diseases.

Although steroids are beneficial to many children with the nephrotic syndrome, other drugs are sometimes necessary. **Cyclophosphamide** is the usual alternative drug, with other, more unusual, drugs being held in reserve. Careful evaluation of any side effects from cyclophosphamide will need to be taken. Toxic effects on the bone marrow can occur as well as possible later infertility. As with all useful but powerful drugs, regular checks on responsiveness and side effects are necessary.

Schooling. After the initial period of hospitalization necessary to put the child on a stable drug and diet regime, it is important that the child's life should return to normal as quickly as possible, with a return to the usual school and activities. School teachers must be made aware of the child's condition and drug and diet regime.

THE FUTURE

As mentioned before, nephrotic syndrome proceeds with periods of relapse and remission. With treatment, the chances of long-term remission is good. Infections should never be treated lightly, however, and special care must be taken at these inevitable times.

SELF-HELP GROUP

National Kidney Foundation
30 East 33rd Street, Suite 1100
New York, NY 10016
800-622-9010 or 212-889-2210
http://www.kidney.org
email: info@kidney.org

Neurofibromatosis

ALTERNATIVE NAME

Von Recklinghausen disease.

INCIDENCE

Neurofibromatosis affects around 1 in every 3,000 live births. The severity of the disease is very variable: some people have only mild symptoms, while others can be severely restricted.

The sexes are affected equally, and there appears to be no predilection for a specific race.

HISTORY

Dr. Friedrich Von Recklinghausen first described the condition in the nineteenth century. He described the main features of neurofibromatosis shown by 90% of sufferers. It was later found that there are certain variations that Dr. Von Recklinghausen did not describe.

CAUSATION

There are two main forms of neurofibromatosis. It is a genetically inherited condition, and in 95% of cases (Nf1), the gene is situated on chromosome 17. The gene for the rarer form (Nf2) is situated on chromosome 22. The condition can be inherited as an autosomal dominant, and there is therefore a 50% chance that the condition will be passed to the children of an affected adult, although it is thought that many cases arise as a new mutation.

CHARACTERISTICS

Nf1

Cafe-au-lait spots: these are coffee-colored patches of skin anywhere on the body. Cafe-au-lait spots are not uncommon among the general population, but people with neurofibromatosis have very many of these patches. The number increases as growth proceeds, and the existing marks become larger. Any child with six or more cafe-au-lait spots should be examined closely for underlying signs of the disorder. By themselves, these cafe-au-lait spots cause no problems (except in a cosmetic sense). The marks are due to an excess of the skin pigment, melanin. Another melanin effect that gives a valuable clue in the diagnosis of neurofibromatosis is a marked freckling of the skin in the armpits of children 10 years old and older with the condition. Occasionally, this freckling is the only sign that the person has the neurofibromatosis gene. (Unfortunately, having this limited condition does not indicate that a person's children will also only have a minor manifestation of the disease. They could be more severely affected.)

Dermal neurofibromatosis: it is this manifestation of the disease that can cause the most problems. These lesions are swellings that appear on the skin on any part of the body. They are not malignant (i.e., they are not cancerous), and they do not spread to other parts of the body. However, they do tend to increase throughout life. Therefore, by the time the sufferer has reached his or her seventies, a great number of these swellings, of all shapes and sizes, may be present. These swellings do not usually make their appearance before puberty. Apart from their disfiguring cosmetic effect, dermal neurofibromata can cause problems when they arise in difficult locations (for example, around the waist, along the neckline, between buttocks, or under shoulder straps). If such problems occur, the growths can be removed surgically, but this procedure does unfortunately cause scarring. If the growths are multiple, they are best left alone. Surgical removal should be left to those swellings that are causing discomfort or irritation.

It is on the basis of the above two signs that the diagnosis of neurofibromatosis is made. There are a few other manifestations that can occur in some cases.

Many people with neurofibromatosis tend to be **shorter than the average.** There is no underlying defect in the bony tissue to account for this condition, and the reason for it is unknown.

Other **skeletal problems** can occur, scoliosis (a sideways curve in the spine) being one of the most common afflictions. Scoliosis usually occurs during the teenage years—the years of maximum growth. Often, no treatment is necessary, as the condition is mild. Swimming is very beneficial for this particular problem, especially in the adolescent years. But if it is more severe, an operation may be required.

Occasionally, the bones of the forearms and legs are thinner than normal, which can result in a bowing of the legs. Fractures can also occur more readily in these thinned bones.

Benign tumors, that is, those that do not spread to other parts of the body, do occur more commonly in neurofibromatosis people than in the general population. These tumors consist of nerve and fibrous tissue (as do the dermal neurofibromata). There are three main sites in the body that can be affected.

- The **spine**—tumors can occur in the nerve roots arising from the spinal cord. The signs and symptoms that arise from a growth of this type will depend on the actual site of the lesion in the spinal cord. Weakness and numbness, and maybe pain, will occur in that part of the body supplied by the affected nerves. If the tumor arises in the lower back region, bladder control can also be affected.
- The **ear**—a tumor arising on the eighth cranial nerve (the nerve associated with hearing) will cause gradual loss of hearing. Vertigo may also occur, as can weakness of the facial muscles on the affected side. (A very rare type of neurofibroma, known as a "central neurofibroma," involves tumors on both auditory nerves. These tumors develop quite independently of each other and can cause bilateral deafness. Sufferers from this rare condition do not usually have cafe-au-lait spots or dermal neurofibromata.)
- The **eye**—the optic nerve can also be the site of a neurofibroma. Signs and symptoms of this condition will include the development of a lazy eye and blurred or double vision.

All these tumors can be removed successfully. Operation is obviously easier if the tumors are small. Therefore, any complaint of deafness, altered vision, or weakness in limbs in a person with neurofibromatosis must be urgently investigated.

Plexiform neurofibromatosis: this type of neurofibroma is exceedingly rare. It consists of complex overgrowths of nervous/fibrous tissue anywhere in the body and can be extensive in size. The most well-known example of this type of neurofibromatosis is the "elephant man," who is thought to have suffered from plexiform neurofibromatosis of the face.

Learning difficulties: there is a slightly higher incidence of reading and writing difficulties in children with neurofibromatosis than in the general population.

Nf2

Cafe-au-lait spots tend to be less than in Nf1, or they may be absent altogether.

Acoustic neuromata—tumors in some part of the hearing system—can occur. These do not usually give rise to problems until the teenage years.

Cataracts can also occur with this form of neurofibromatosis.

MANAGEMENT IMPLICATIONS

Dermal neurofibromata: watch must be kept on the development of new swellings, especially in problem sites. Treatment consists of surgical removal of swellings that give rise to irritation or pressure problems. Regular follow-up is ideal.

Deafness and **visual problems** such as lazy eye or blurred vision must be investigated promptly. Accurate diagnosis of the cause, followed by appropriate treatment, is essential.

Genetic counseling should be given as the child approaches maturity. Difficult decisions will need to be taken regarding the birth of children.

Blood pressure should be monitored regularly, as there is a higher incidence of both a specific tumor of the adrenal gland (pheochromocytoma) and also the narrowing of the renal artery among persons with neurofibromatosis. Both of these conditions will give rise to raised blood pressure.

Nonaccidental injury: investigators will need to remember the increased risk of fractures of the long bones.

Emotional problems associated with neurofibromatosis must not be overlooked. Adolescents are especially concerned regarding skin blemishes, and the first appearance of dermal neurofibromata at this time of life can be traumatic. Parents, too, need support. Their "guilt" regarding the genetic inheritance of the disease can be very real.

Learning difficulties of a moderate degree can affect neurofibromatosis children to a slightly greater extent than the general population. Falling behind in school work should alert teachers to the child's possible need for special help. Appropriate schooling will prevent the development of the secondary behavioral problems that arise as a result of frustration and apparent failure in academic subjects. Absences from school, on occasions, may have a deleterious effect on some children's education. Surgical removal of dermal neurofibromata may cause the child to need in-patient treatment for variable lengths of time. Home schooling, or work sent home, may need to be arranged at these times.

SELF-HELP GROUPS

Neurofibromatosis, Inc.
8855 Annapolis Road, Suite 110
Lanham, MD 20706-2924
301-577-8984
http://www.nfinc.org
email: nfinc1@aol.com

National Neurofibromatosis Foundation
95 Pine Street, 16th Floor
New York, NY 10005
212-344-6633
http://www.nf.org
email: nnff@nf.org

Niemann–Pick Disease

ALTERNATIVE NAMES

Sphingomyelinase deficiency (sea-blue histiocyte disease).

INCIDENCE

There are 4 types of Niemann–Pick Disease: A, B, C, and D, which all have an accumulation of sphingomyelin in various tissues of the body as the basic defect. This accumulation is due to a deficiency of the enzyme sphingomyelinase, which normally breaks down that lipid substance. Type A is the most common, and severe, variant, and it occurs mainly in people of Ashkenazi Jewish descent. All types may vary in severity and, therefore, prognosis (see below).

Niemann–Pick disease is a rare disorder; the actual number of cases is not recorded. Both sexes can be affected. Prenatal diagnosis is possible for types A and B and for most forms of type C.

HISTORY

The type D variant is closely allied to type C. It has been traced back to a seventeenth century French Acadian couple from Nova Scotia. There is a fifth variant known by the splendid name of "sea-blue histiocyte disease." The name refers to a preponderance of particular cells found in the bone marrow that are of a foamy—or "sea-blue"—appearance. These cells can also be seen in other types of Niemann–Pick disease.

A new classification is being created to replace the rather confused typing in current use.

CAUSATION

Niemann–Pick disease is inherited as an autosomal recessive disorder.

CHARACTERISTICS

Type A

Type A Niemann–Pick disease shows up early in life—within the first few months—with an **enlarged abdomen** (cf. Gaucher disease) due to the enlargement of the liver and spleen. The baby will fail to **gain weight** adequately, and **developmental progress** will be slow.

Skin may be a yellowish-brown color with little subcutaneous fat. This latter fact, together with the lack of weight gain. leads to a starved, almost emaciated appearance.

Many of these babies, when their eyes are examined with an ophthalmoscope, have a **cherry-red spot** on a particular part of the retina.

Regretfully, due to the accumulation of lipid material in various organs of the body, including the lungs, children with this type of Niemann–Pick disease will die within the first three years of life.

Type B

Type B Niemann–Pick disease usually becomes apparent early in childhood when the **enlarged abdomen** is observed, although it may be early adulthood before milder cases of the condition are noticed. The swollen abdomen is due to abnormal deposits of unmetabolized sphingomyelin in the liver and the spleen.

Infiltration of sphingomyelin into the **lungs** can be the presenting feature, with infection and general respiratory difficulties alerting parents to potential problems.

Most children will feel generally **unwell,** and there will be poor **growth** and general health.

In this type of Niemann–Pick disease, **developmental delay** is less marked than with type A, and there appears to be no direct involvement of the central nervous system.

Life span can be normal for those people with a later onset of the disease.

Type C

With this type, onset of symptoms can vary widely from being obvious in the very early days of life through to symptoms only becoming apparent in early adulthood.

Symptoms of **abdominal swelling** can occur along with general symptoms of ill-health and a failure to thrive.

Central nervous system symptoms occur as time passes, with **general development** being progressively delayed. **Ataxia** and **seizures** are not uncommon. Poor muscular control (accounting for the ataxia) can cause **speech difficulties.**

Regretfully, many children will die in the teenage years.

Type D

Type D Niemann–Pick disease, or the Nova Scotia variant, is very similar to type C. Life expectancy is much reduced, and affected children rarely reach 20 years of age.

INVESTIGATIONS

Bone marrow testing will show the cells specific to the disease. Analysis of samples from the liver and/or spleen will also show the typical storage pattern.

MANAGEMENT IMPLICATIONS

Although there is presently no specific treatment for children with this type of abnormal storage disease, parents and care givers will need much support in making life as normal as possible for the child with Niemann–Pick disease.

Regular **developmental testing** is necessary to determine the level of the child's abilities. This sort of test is especially important for children with the types of Niemann–Pick disease in which life span can be expected beyond the first decade.

In cases of recurrent **lung** infection, seen most frequently in type B, early prescription of antibiotics is vital.

Anticonvulsant drugs may also need to be prescribed if seizures are a part of the symptomatology.

Removal of the **spleen** may be a necessary procedure in some cases if this organ is grossly—and uncomfortably—overloaded and swollen with excess sphingomyelin.

Schooling will need to be geared to the child's specific difficulties, and regular review of the child's progress will need to be made. It must also be remembered that the frequent bouts of illness and possible hospital admissions can further reduce educational benefits.

THE FUTURE

The future can vary greatly from individual to individual, depending upon the type of Niemann–Pick disease and its severity. Unfortunately, in only a relatively minority of cases will life expectancy be good.

SELF-HELP GROUP

National Niemann–Pick Disease Foundation
3734 East Olive Avenue
Gilbert, AZ 85234-3117
602-497-6638
http://www.nnpdf.org
email: stevekenyon@netwrx.net

Noonan Syndrome

INCIDENCE

Noonan syndrome is thought to occur in between 1 in every 1,000 and 1 in every 2,500 births. Diagnosis can be difficult because the syndrome has a number of features that vary both among individuals and with time. For example, the facial features that at birth are characteristic of Noonan syndrome, may alter greatly by the time adult life is reached. Also, a sign that is obvious in one individual with the syndrome may be absent in another. It is thought that there may be some adults who have Noonan syndrome, but who are undiagnosed due to lack of widespread knowledge about the syndrome; therefore, the incidence of the condition may be greater than originally thought. Both sexes can be affected.

HISTORY

In 1963, Dr. Jacqueline Noonan, a pediatric cardiologist, first reported the close association of a specific heart defect with short stature and an unusual facial appearance.

CAUSATION

Noonan syndrome is a genetic disorder passed on as an autosomal dominant, but it can be, and often is, a sporadic occurrence. There is no specific test, at present, either clinical or biochemical, that can aid diagnosis. Therefore, the association of specific physical characteristics is of prime importance in the recognition of Noonan syndrome.

At present, there is no prenatal test for Noonan syndrome, but ultrasound scanning early in pregnancy may be able to pick up some of the cardiac abnormalities.

Genetic counseling of parents—and brothers and sisters when they reach reproductive age—is advisable following the birth of a child with Noonan syndrome.

It is thought that Noonan syndrome may have a close genetic association with Turner syndrome, as many of the characteristics of the two syndromes are similar.

CHARACTERISTICS

There are three main features that characterize Noonan syndrome. Other features are often also present and can help confirm the diagnosis, but these are variable both in degree and their presence in each individual.

Congenital heart defects are diagnosable at birth. The defects can be any one or more of the following, although not all these defects will be found in any one child.

- **Pulmonary stenosis,** in which the valve in the pulmonary artery is narrowed or poorly formed. This is the most common of the heart defects.
- **Atrial septal defect:** this is a defect in the wall between the two upper chambers of the heart.
- **Ventricular septal defect:** this is a defect in the wall of the heart between the two ventricles.

Symptoms relating to these cardiac problems will vary according to the type, and degree, of abnormality. Many children who have been found on routine examination to have a defect will not need treatment and will be able to live a normal life; others will need drugs and/or cardiac surgery for their condition.

Short stature: this is not extreme, as in some of the other syndromes (cf. Turner syndrome or achondroplasia, for example). Children with Noonan syndrome tend to be at the lower end of the growth range, around the tenth percentile. Special charts are currently being prepared for use with children with Noonan syndrome. These are necessary because "normal" height gain is not relevant for children with this syndrome, whose growth is along different lines. Bodily proportions are correct. Final height—an important factor when discussing the future—can be estimated from serial measurements on appropriate growth charts.

Facial characteristics, as mentioned, are seen in varying degree in each individual with Noonan syndrome. Also, as the child matures, the distinctive features tend to become less noticeable. Some of the most obvious characteristics are as follows.

- **Eyes** are widely spaced and tend to be large with a downward slant. There is also frequently a ptosis (drooping of the eyelids), which persists throughout life.
- The **neck** tends to be short with a low hair-line and loose folds of skin in the nape of the neck. (This latter characteristic is also reminiscent of Turner syndrome.)

- **Ears** tend to be low-set and have distinctive lobes that are bent forwards.
- The **nose** frequently has a flattened bridge.

These three main groups of signs—cardiac problems, short stature, and specific facial features—make up the major characteristics of Noonan syndrome. There can be other associated features, such as the following.

Poor muscle tone, which can give rise to poor sucking in the early months, may be a concern. Mild degrees of clumsiness throughout childhood are often seen, leading to, for example, problems playing sports and a tendency to bump into objects.

Undescended testes occur more frequently than usual. Testes can also be small, and infertility may pose problems when the reproductive years are reached.

Intelligence levels are wide ranging, but specific learning difficulties can be encountered, especially when the child is learning to speak. Children with Noonan syndrome tend to mature late and often prefer to play with children younger than themselves.

Occasionally, a mild **hearing loss** is present, and it is important that doctors check for this condition throughout childhood.

It must be stressed that many of these characteristics are to be found also in the general childhood population. It is only when a number of these occur together that Noonan syndrome can be confidently diagnosed.

MANAGEMENT IMPLICATIONS

Heart defects diagnosed at birth, or subsequently, must be checked on a regular basis by a pediatric cardiologist. Treatment—with drugs and/or cardiac surgery—may be necessary in a small number of children.

Feeding difficulties, which can occur during the early months of life due to poor muscle tone, may need special sympathetic help from staff both in the hospital and in the community. With severe feeding problems, which occur rarely, nasogastric feeding may be necessary for a short time in the neonatal period. Vomiting can also be a feature of Noonan syndrome. It can be projectile in character, and differential diagnosis from hypertrophic pyloric stenosis is necessary under these circumstances. These feeding difficulties usually resolve themselves within the first few months of life.

Growth must be monitored regularly throughout childhood. Treatment with growth hormone for children who are growing slowly has been tried, but results are yet to be evaluated. Lack of inches and the tendency to immaturity will need to be understood by childcare workers and, later, by teachers. It is all too easy to underestimate a child's potential ability by treating him/her as younger than his/her chronological age.

Undescended testes: if this problem is present, it will need surgical intervention before school age is reached, both to ensure the best chance of fertility and to reduce the chance of malignant change.

Speech, vision, and **hearing problems,** which are all marginally more common in children with Noonan syndrome, will need specific help and treatment. Speech therapy in particular is often indicated for articulation and language delay. Lazy eye and myopia will need appropriate care and correction, as will any hearing loss due to secretory otitis media.

Genetic counseling is advisable for members of the family who have a child diagnosed with Noonan syndrome.

THE FUTURE

Children with Noonan syndrome usually lead absolutely normal lives. In relatively few cases, cardiac defects need treatment. Severe instances of this aspect of Noonan syndrome may restrict life expectancy. Shortness of stature is an irritant rather than a severe problem.

SELF-HELP GROUP

Noonan Syndrome Support Group
P.O. Box 145
Upperco, MD 21155
888-686-2224 or 410-374-5245
http://www.noonansyndrome.org
email: info@noonansyndrome.org

Ollier Disease

ALTERNATIVE NAMES

Ollier syndrome; enchondromatosis.

INCIDENCE

The incidence of Ollier disease is not exactly known. Either sex can be affected.

CAUSATION

At present, there is no known genetic inheritance concerned with Ollier disease—all cases arising spontaneously. The basic defect is in the cartilage at the growing ends of the long straight bones of the body. These bones include the bones of the hands as well as the longer arm and leg bones.

There is no known prenatal diagnosis at present.

CHARACTERISTICS

Ollier disease is characterized by **swellings in the bones** of many parts of the body, which are caused by the overgrowth of cartilage in these positions. When the legs are affected, there can be **bowing of the legs** as well as some **shortening** of the affected limb. The latter is results from cartilage interfering in normal bone growth. On the hands, bony swellings become obvious as the mass of cartilaginous cells enlarge.

There is no definitive pattern in these bony growths, and any of the long bones of the body can be affected in a random fashion. The condition can be confined to one or two bones, or it can result in generalized deformity in many parts of the body. Fortunately, the bones of the head and spine are not involved in this pathological process.

Ollier disease can be recognized in infancy, but diagnosis is more frequently made after the age of around 2 years. At this age, the normal rapid growth will bring to light uneven developments in the bony skeleton. Some children with this condition will experience **pain** at times of maximum growth.

No other system in the body is involved in Ollier disease. It is important that this condition is clearly distinguished form a similar condition known as **Maffucci syndrome.** In this latter syndrome, there are many hemangiomas (red nevi of varying size) present all over the body. The prognosis for this syndrome is more serious than for Ollier disease, as there is a far greater chance that Maffucci syndrome will involve malignant changes in the bony lesions.

There is a tendency to **fracture** of the long bones in Ollier disease. This occurrence may be the first sign of the presence of the condition

Short stature can occur if the long bones of the legs are severely affected. As growth slows, so does the development of new cartilaginous lesions. The lesions already present ossify and become hard.

MANAGEMENT IMPLICATIONS

Many children with Ollier disease will lead perfectly normal lives if only a few bones are affected. It is when growth is inhibited or asymmetric that problems can arise, such as:

- **Physical activities** at school, for example, can be more difficult for children with this condition.
- **Fractures** can occur with greater readiness than for children with normal bones. (Care must be taken to exclude Ollier disease in cases of suspected child abuse.)
- **Pain,** especially during periods of active growth, can occur. Pain will need to be treated with analgesic drugs while it persists.
- **Schooling** can be in mainstream institutions, as there is no intellectual impairment with this condition. Teachers should be informed of the reason for the—sometimes very obvious—swellings on their pupil's hands, legs, and arms. They should also be warned of possible periods of pain and the possibility of fractures following minimal trauma.

Orthopedic intervention may be needed in cases of severe deformity. Care must be taken to exclude malignant change in any of the bony lesions, although such lesions are rare in this disease. X-ray examination is necessary if the bony changes become painful and enlarge rapidly.

THE FUTURE

The expected life span for a sufferer from Ollier disease is normal. Malignant changes in the bones are rare, but must always be remembered. Genetic counseling is advisable before pregnancy is embarked upon.

SELF-HELP GROUP

Ollier/Maffucci Self-Help Group
1824 Millwood Road
Sumter, SC 29150
803-775-1757
http://uhsweb.edu/olliers/olliers.htm
email: Olliers@aol.com

Osteogenesis Imperfecta

ALTERNATIVE NAMES

Brittle bone disease; Lobstein syndrome.

INCIDENCE

"Brittle bone disease" is a rare disorder; the number of babies born with the condition being around 3 to 4 per 100,000. There appear to be four distinct types of osteogenesis imperfecta, and the incidence varies slightly with each type.

Type 1 is the most common form found in most populations, although type 3 is more frequently found in South Africa among the black population. Type 2 is usually so severe that most babies with this manifestation of brittle bone disease are stillborn or die in the first few weeks of life. Type 4 is similar to type 1, the main difference being that in type 4, the "whites" of the eyes do not show the characteristic blue coloration of type 1.

Children of all races can be affected, and there is no distinction in the incidence rates of boys and girls.

Type 1, being the most frequently seen manifestation of this rare condition, will be described.

CAUSATION

Osteogenesis imperfecta is a genetic disease that is inherited as an autosomal dominant. New mutations account for a number of babies with the condition. Biochemically, there is found to be a defect in the production of one of the precursors of collagen, a substance closely involved in skeletal make-up. At present, there is no specific prenatal test, although severe cases can be detected by ultrasound scanning.

CHARACTERISTICS

Skeletal changes: all bones, but in particular those of the arms and legs, are especially fragile and prone to fractures after a minimal amount of injury. Toddlers, who fall frequently as they learn to walk, are especially prone to such fractures. Most children with brittle bone disease will have had at least one fracture before they reach five years of age.

Spinal deformities, including both kyphosis and scoliosis, can occur later in life, but such deformities rarely occur during childhood. In adults, spinal abnormalities can result in a loss of height.

Eyes: children with type 1 osteogenesis imperfecta have a marked blue color to the sclera (the white part) of their eyes. This unusual coloration persists throughout life, and it is a consistent aid to diagnosis of type 1 osteogenesis imperfecta. People with type 4 often have blue sclera at birth, but the color gradually fades, until by the time adulthood is reached, eyes look completely normal. Vision is not affected by this manifestation.

Teeth: type 1 is further divided into two distinct subgroups, one group having specific abnormalities of the teeth. These children have teeth that are a yellowish-brown color. Teeth are of normal size and shape, but they can be easily cracked or broken, and they must be watched for decay due to excessive wear.

Hearing can be impaired in children with osteogenesis imperfecta. A conductive type of hearing loss, due to deformity in the small bones (ossicles) in the middle ear, is most usual. Sensory hearing loss can also occur in addition to the conductive loss, high frequency tones being most frequently lost.

Blood vessels are often excessively fragile, so that in addition to frequent fracture on minimal injury, bruising also occurs relatively easily.

MANAGEMENT IMPLICATIONS

Skeletal system: the peak ages for fractures is between 2 and 3 years, and again between 10 and 15 years old. These two peaks coincide with the periods of greatest activity in the growing child's life. When fractures occur, they must be appropriately treated, making sure that the long bones are carefully realigned so that permanent disability does not result. Physical therapy is often needed after a fracture has healed so that resultant deformity is minimized. Orthopedic advice on the possibility of procedures to stabilize limbs that have been subjected to repeated fractures is very worthwhile. Rods positioned inside long bones may be considered if fractures are very frequent. Protective splinting of the long bones can be necessary.

It is of vital importance in possible cases of child abuse that the diagnosis of osteogenesis imperfecta is known, as the easily fractured limbs and excessive bruising associated with the condition can be confused with signs of abuse.

Teeth must receive ongoing and adequate dental care. Advanced dental techniques can change the yellow color of some children's teeth to a more attractive color.

Hearing must be assessed at regular intervals, and hearing aids supplied if necessary.

Schooling: mainstream schooling is the norm for children with brittle bone disease, except for those children who are very severely affected. Teachers must be informed of their pupil's condition, so that they can act appropriately and quickly should any injury be sustained during school hours. Body-contact sports should be avoided due to the risk of fractures on minimal injury.

It can be difficult to strike a balance between protecting the child from injury and allowing him/her to lead a normal life. As the child with osteogenesis imperfecta matures, she/he will learn which activities to avoid.

Occupational therapy for severely affected children can give insight into suitable and practical activities.

Trials with **calcitonin** and **fluoride** are presently being undertaken in an endeavor to reduce the number of fractures suffered by children with osteogenesis imperfecta.

Counseling in the adolescent years is of importance so that the young person has an understanding of his/her genetic condition and the care that he/she should take in the future.

THE FUTURE

A normal life span can be expected in the vast majority of people with osteogenesis imperfecta, often with very few problems due to their inherited condition.

Careers with minimal physical contact should be chosen in order to avoid fractures.

Pregnancy can pose problems for severely affected women. The hormonal changes occurring at that time increase laxity of ligaments and so predispose the bones to fractures from even minimal trauma. Cesarean section is often considered a wise mode of delivery.

SELF-HELP GROUPS

Osteogenesis Imperfecta Foundation
804 West Diamond Avenue, Suite 210
Gaithersburg, MD 20878
301-947-0083
http://www.oif.org
email: bonelink@aol.com

Children's Brittle Bone Foundation
P.O. Box 27
Highland Park, IL 60035
847-433-4981

Patau Syndrome

ALTERNATIVE NAMES

Trisomy D; trisomy 13 syndrome.

INCIDENCE

The incidence of Patau syndrome is reportedly between 1 in 6,000 and 1 in 8,000 births.

There is a slightly higher preponderance of boys being born with this syndrome. Due to the multiple, and severe, malformations associated with this condition, between 80% and 90% of the babies born alive with this syndrome die within the first few months of life. Regretfully, those children who do survive are severely handicapped.

Patau syndrome has been reported all over the world.

Chorionic villus sampling, between 9 and 12 weeks of pregnancy, and/or amniocentesis, at 16 weeks of pregnancy, can detect this syndrome prenatally. Ultrasound can detect the decreased size of the head in a baby with Patau syndrome.

There is some evidence to suggest that older mothers are more likely to give birth to a child with this syndrome. Paternal age does not appear to have any effect.

HISTORY

This syndrome was first described and classified by Patau in 1960. In 1984, further research into the genetics of the condition were undertaken in an European study.

CAUSATION

Patau syndrome is a chromosomal disorder in which, as the alternative name trisomy 13 syndrome implies, there are 3 chromosomes in the 13 position (cf. Down syndrome or trisomy 21). As with both Down and Edwards syndromes, the total chromosome count is 47 instead of the normal 46.

A "mosaic" trisomy 13 can occasionally occur. Under these circumstances, not all of the baby's cells have the abnormal 47 chromosomes;

some cells have the normal complement of 46 chromosomes. Boys or girls with this genetic make-up will be less severely affected; they probably account for most of the children who survive infancy.

CHARACTERISTICS

Characteristics are multiple and severe. Only the most severely affected babies show all the abnormalities, but 100% of babies with Patau syndrome are mentally retarded, and they all have varying degrees of muscular abnormalities. Boys also have undescended testes. These findings alone do not, of course, enable the diagnosis of Patau syndrome to be made. The added problems that can occur are:

- **Microcephaly** is present in a high proportion of cases and can be detected prenatally by ultrasound.
- **cleft palate and/or lip** can frequently occur;
- **extra fingers** may be an obvious feature, as is a single palmar crease.

Those three features are the ones most commonly associated with this syndrome, but the following characteristics can also occur:

- The baby's **eyes** can be small, together with a small lower jaw.
- The baby's **neck** can be short, with folds of extra surplus skin at the nape.
- Defects in the **bones of the skull** may be present. (This feature is rarely found in other chromosomal disorders, and it therefore can be of assistance in the diagnosis of Patau syndrome before the chromosomal analysis has been reported.)
- **Heart defects** of several different types are a frequent feature, as are **renal abnormalities.** These severe, and often fatal, defects are frequently only discovered at postmortem examination.

A number of other abnormalities, such as defects in the spine, abdomen, or sex organs, can also occur. The severity and site of such abnormalities varies from baby to baby.

INVESTIGATIONS

To confirm the clinical diagnosis of Patau syndrome, a chromosomal analysis of the baby's cells must be done. Further investigations into possible cardiac and renal defects will need to be done as problems relating to these systems present themselves in the early, difficult days of life.

MANAGEMENT IMPLICATIONS

In the very early days of life, **feeding** can be a problem due to both the poor muscle tone and the smallness of the lower jaw found in many babies. If a cleft palate/lip is present, feeding problems are worsened.

If the baby survives the early days of life, routine **developmental checks** will need to be done to determine the extent of the mental handicap, which is usually severe.

Heart and renal defects will need medical intervention as they become apparent.

The **cleft palate/lip,** too, will need surgical attention as soon as the baby's general condition is stable enough to withstand the necessary treatment.

Parents will need much **support,** physical help, and encouragement to cope with their child's many and severe handicaps. Due to the expected short life span of the majority of children with this syndrome, preparation for the baby's death must also be a factor in the forefront of the minds of the people caring for the family.

Bereavement counseling must not be forgotten following the death of the child.

Genetic counseling is also advisable before parents pursue a further pregnancy, as some cases do arise from a specific translocation.

THE FUTURE

The future is bleak for babies born with Patau syndrome. Ninety-five percent of the affected babies die by the age of 3 years, and survivors are severely handicapped, both mentally and physically.

SELF-HELP GROUP

SOFT USA
2982 South Union Street
Rochester, NY 14624
716-594-4621 or 800-716-7638
http://www.trisomy.org
email: barb@trisomy.org

Phenylketonuria

ALTERNATIVE NAMES

Folling disease; hyperphenylalaninemia; phenylalanine hydroxylase deficiency.

INCIDENCE

The incidence of phenylketonuria is between 1 in 10,000 and 1 in 15,000 live births. This condition is found more frequently in Caucasian populations and rarely occurs among black or Ashkenazi Jewish people. People with phenylketonuria are typically fair-haired and blue-eyed, although there may be a few exceptions to this observation.

Both sexes are equally affected by the disease.

There is no routine prenatal diagnosis in current use, but new techniques are being researched for this purpose and for the detection of carriers of the condition. A test is performed routinely on all newborn babies that detects the abnormality at a very early stage.

CAUSATION

Phenylketonuria is caused by the deficiency of a certain vital enzyme (phenylalanine hydroxylase—PAH) that is necessary for the conversion of phenylalanine into tyrosine. As a result of this defect, there is a build-up of phenylalanine (which is an essential amino acid) in the blood. It is the excess of this substance that gives rise to the signs and symptoms of the disease.

Phenylketonuria is inherited in an autosomal recessive manner.

CHARACTERISTICS

The enzyme block to the normal metabolism of phenylalanine causes this amino acid to build up in the tissues of the body; the condition will have long-lasting and severe effects if it is not controlled by an appropriate diet. A certain amount of phenylalanine is necessary for proper growth, so the diet must be very carefully controlled during the growing years.

If the condition is not diagnosed at birth, the following effects will occur over the weeks and months after birth:

- **mental retardation,** of a moderate to a severe degree, will be the inevitable result of untreated phenylketonuria;
- in the early days of life, severe **vomiting,** and occasionally **seizures** can occur;
- the baby's **skin** can be dry, with an eczematous rash also noticeable;
- it has been said that children with untreated phenylketonuria have a "mousy" smell. The odor is due to phenylacetic acid (which is present in excess because of the lack of the appropriate metabolic enzyme) excreted in the sweat and the urine;
- expected life span may be shortened.

It must be emphasized that the above characteristics only occur when this condition is untreated. With the appropriate dietary care, the outlook for intelligence and life span is excellent.

MANAGEMENT IMPLICATIONS

The initial **blood test** done within the first few days of life to detect the condition is vitally important. Of equal importance in the prevention of mental handicap is the early commencement of an appropriate **diet.** A special nutritional regimen must definitely begin before the baby is one month of age, preferably sooner.

There is an intermediate form of this condition—known as hyperphenylalaninemia—in which the levels of phenylalanine are raised but not dangerously so. It is thought that this form is a less severe expression of phenylketonuria, with perhaps only a relative lack of the appropriate enzyme dealing with the metabolism of this amino acid.

Alternatively, the raised phenylalanine levels may occur transitory during the first 3 months of life. A possible explanation of this feature is a delayed maturation of this specific enzyme system. Skilled analysis and follow-up is needed to differentiate between phenylketonuria and these connected conditions.

The **diet** for children with phenylketonuria is not especially palatable, but with advice from a dietitian, children will accept it. In infancy, specially prepared infant formulas are necessary. Because a certain amount of phenylalanine is vital for growth, this amino acid must not be omitted altogether from the diet. It is given in measured amounts in the diet, with frequent checks on blood levels. Foods with a low phenylalanine level (flour, pasta, cookies, etc.) can be obtained on prescription. A strict diet is usually recommended until the child is at least 10 years old.

Some relaxation of the diet after that age is possible, but blood levels of phenylalanine must still be frequently checked.

Schooling will offer no problem on the intellectual level, but school staff must be aware of the dietary restrictions so vital to the health and well-being of the child with phenylketonuria.

Adolescence can be an especially difficult time, when rebellion against the restrictive diet can, understandably, occur. Support and sympathy from dietitians and other care givers is necessary during those formative years.

THE FUTURE

If the diet is followed, the outlook for children with phenylketonuria is excellent for both life span and intellectual ability.

Special care will need to be taken during pregnancy. Babies born to mothers with phenylketonuria stand a greater risk of brain damage due to the woman's high phenylalanine levels. This damage can occur during the very early days of pregnancy. Specialist advice should, therefore, be taken well before pregnancy begins, so that diet can be adjusted to fully stabilize the amount of phenylalanine in the woman's blood.

SELF-HELP GROUPS

Children's PKU Network
1520 State Street, Suite 110
San Diego, CA 92101
619-233-3202

PKU CORPS
Children's Hospital
300 Longwood Avenue
Boston, MA 02115
617-355-7346
email: PKU@A1.tch.harvard.edu

Pierre–Robin Syndrome

ALTERNATIVE NAME

Robin anomaly.

INCIDENCE

Pierre–Robin syndrome is a rare condition, which can cause severe problems in infancy. It can exist on its own, or as part of a wider group of rare syndromes, all of which have the Pierre–Robin anomaly in addition to other features. Classification of these other syndromes is, at present, unclear.

CAUSATION

The inheritance pattern of Pierre–Robin syndrome is not exactly known. There is a possibility that the condition may be inherited as an autosomal recessive. There have also been suggestions that there may be an X-linked variant that has the additional problems of heart abnormalities and clubfeet.

It is presumed that both boys and girls are affected equally, apart from, of course, the X-linked variety.

There is no prenatal diagnosis possible, although the cleft palate or the small jaw may be seen on ultrasound.

CHARACTERISTICS

The features of Pierre–Robin syndrome are confined to the lower part of the face and mouth. The initial abnormality from which all the other features follow is a very **under-developed lower jaw.**

During the process of development, the baby's **palate** frequently has a rounded cleft in its length.

Because of the initial defect, the baby can have severe **breathing problems** at birth. The small lower jaw causes the tongue to be positioned further back than is usual. As a result of these unusual anatomical features, the baby's tongue will be prone to fall back into his/her throat, thereby effectively obstructing breathing (cf. Treacher Collins syndrome, but in that condition, the abnormality is not as severe as in Pierre–Robin syndrome).

Swallowing difficulties, again due to the positioning of the tongue, can cause problems with feeding in the early days.

Once the difficulties of breathing and feeding in the early days of life are over, the baby's lower jaw will fortunately develop into a normal size in relation to the rest of his/her face. This "catch-up" growth is especially marked during the first two years of life.

Later on in childhood, there may be **dental problems** with overcrowding and irregular teeth in the lower jaw.

Very rarely, some mild degree of **mental handicap** may develop, due to oxygen lack in the first few weeks of life when breathing difficulties are at their worst.

Pierre–Robin syndrome is an interesting example of how one, comparatively mild, abnormality can have a number of additional effects that have far-reaching influences.

MANAGEMENT IMPLICATIONS

Breathing difficulties will mean that the baby will need intensive care facilities for the first few weeks of life. It is advisable that all newborn babies with Pierre–Robin syndrome should lay in a partially prone position. (The completely prone position should be avoided due to its possible link with sudden infant death syndrome. In the intensive care nursery, babies are monitored continually and immediate action can be taken should any problems arise.) This position will allow the baby's tongue to fall forward, rather than backwards into his/her throat, and so avoids obstruction to breathing. Intubation facilities should always be immediately available in the newborn period for babies with Pierre–Robin syndrome.

Feeding difficulties will also need special care in the early days. Simple measures such as feeding the baby in an upright position may be all that is necessary to ensure adequate nutrition.

If a **cleft palate** is present, as is often the case, it will complicate the feeding of the baby. A modified nipple and/or a temporary dental plate can initially help with feeding. The cleft palate will need surgery to close the gap and ensure easier feeding, breathing, and speech. Surgery is often delayed until around three or four years of age to allow maximum possible growth of the palate toward the midline. Once the early problems are over, the baby with Pierre–Robin syndrome will develop along completely normal lines.

A few extra problems may arise later in childhood, again all arising from the small lower jaw.

Speech therapy may be necessary in the preschool years to ensure clear speech following the repair of the cleft palate.

Dental care must be given throughout the early years, until all the secondary teeth have erupted satisfactorily. Orthodontic treatment may be needed to straighten crooked teeth and to ensure a correct "bite."

In very rare cases, special educational facilities will be needed for children with reduced **intellectual ability.** Mental retardation is possible if the breathing difficulties have been very severe in infancy, but it is by no means inevitable. The vast majority of children with Pierre–Robin syndrome will have the same abilities and physical development as their peers during the school years.

THE FUTURE

Most children with Pierre–Robin syndrome will grow into adults with the same range of abilities and aptitudes as every one else. The difficulties in the early days of life will only very rarely have any long-lasting effects.

Genetic counseling is advisable before a pregnancy is embarked upon.

SELF-HELP GROUPS

Pierre Robin Network
P.O. Box 3274
Quincy, IL 62305
http://www.pierrerobin.org
email: prn@pierrerobin.org

FACES: The National Craniofacial Association
P.O. Box 11082
Chattanooga, TN 37401
423-266-1632
http://www.faces~cranio.org
email: faces@faces~cranio.org

Prader–Willi Syndrome

ALTERNATIVE NAME

Prader–Labhart–Willi syndrome.

INCIDENCE

The precise incidence of Prader–Willi Syndrome is not known, but it is thought to be around 1 in every 15,000 live births. It is a rare disorder, affecting both sexes equally. There are probably a number of older people who have Prader–Willi syndrome who are undiagnosed due to the lack of knowledge in the past regarding the characteristic features of the condition.

HISTORY

Dr. Langdon Down (who also described Down syndrome) described the syndrome, which he termed "polysardia," in 1887. The characteristics of Prader–Willi syndrome were documented by three doctors—Prader, Willi, and Labhart in 1956.

CAUSATION

The mode of inheritance of Prader–Willi syndrome is uncertain. About 50% of sufferers have been shown to have a small deletion on the long arm of chromosome 15, while other sufferers appear to have a normal chromosome pattern.

There is a connection between this syndrome and Angelman syndrome, in which there is also, in a percentage of cases, a deletion or rearrangement on the long arm of chromosome 15. The parent from which the abnormality is inherited apparently determines which of these syndromes occurs. Prader–Willi syndrome appears to be derived from the father.

It is not possible, at present, to diagnose the condition prenatally.

CHARACTERISTICS

Hypotonia is commonly seen at birth in babies with Prader–Willi syndrome. This condition gradually improves over the months and years. Babies with this syndrome are often born in a breech position, which possibly has something to do with the hypotonia of the baby. Because of the relative weakness of their muscles, children and adults with Prader–Willi syndrome tend to have difficulties with coordination and balance throughout life.

Sucking proves a problem due to poor muscle tone, and it frequently causes feeding difficulties during the first months of life. As a result of these problems, the baby can fail to thrive adequately during the first year of life. Other reasons for failure to thrive must also, of course, be checked out.

An **insatiable appetite,** in contradistinction from the early failure to thrive, makes its appearance between the ages of two and four years. This appetite develops into an obsessive eating pattern, and, unless controlled, can result in gross obesity. The onset of this hearty appetite may be one of the first clues pointing to the diagnosis of Prader–Willi syndrome. This trait is thought to be due to some abnormality in the specific part of the brain concerned with appetite control. The obesity that often ensues is particularly hard to treat, and behavior problems can result from attempts to control food intake.

Short stature, with small hands and feet, is a common feature of Prader–Willi syndrome. This reduction in size can be seen on prenatal scans.

Sexual development is limited, particularly in boys with Prader–Willi syndrome. The penis and scrotum are small and underdeveloped. No man or woman with Prader–Willi syndrome has been known to have children.

Learning disability of a moderate degree is the general rule, although 10% of children with Prader–Willi syndrome have a normal IQ. Children with Prader–Willi syndrome are usually outgoing and affectionate, but they can have outbursts of rage or temper tantrums, particularly in situations involving eating. These outbursts are short-lived, but they can be difficult to control. The best method is to try to manipulate known situations that provoke outbursts. Moods can swing in the opposite direction—to those of exuberant joy—which can be almost as difficult to contain. Again, situation manipulation is the best method to employ to control this difficulty.

Seizures can occasionally occur, and EEG tracings can be abnormal. Seizures are not a common feature, but they are one that must always be remembered.

MANAGEMENT IMPLICATIONS

Feeding difficulties during the first year of life will need expert help. Breastfeeding for the first few months is to be encouraged if at all possible. Small, frequent feeds, whether of breast milk or formula, will improve weight gain, and ensure that the small, hypotonic baby with Prader–Willi syndrome does not tire.

Other, more usual, causes of failure to thrive must be excluded, and remedied if found to be present.

The **insatiable appetite** can cause great problems when it appears around the toddler years. After the feeding problems experienced earlier, parents will be only too delighted that their child is eating well! But as excessive weight becomes a problem, a strict dietary regime will be more readily accepted. It is wise to involve a professional dietitian to ensure that adequate nutrients are taken for growth and development while keeping excess weight gain under control. This aspect of the condition can be one of the most difficult to manage, especially in the younger age group.

Learning disability, if present, is generally moderate, although it can be severe, IQs ranging from 20 to 80. Special schooling will be necessary for some children. A regular, sheltered lifestyle with maximum encouragement and understanding should be the aim in the care of children with Prader–Willi syndrome. As few affected children will be able to lead an independent life, it is important that appropriate skills training is given from as early an age as possible. Special skills in reading and other visual organizational skills (such as the ability to easily solve jigsaw puzzles quickly) are often found in children with Prader–Willi syndrome.

Difficulties with **coordination** and **balance** will need to be considered during schooling and training. The help of a physical therapist is helpful to maximize muscle strength and use.

Scoliosis can be a problem in adolescence, unless muscle tone is strengthened, and it may need orthopedic treatment.

Severe behavioral problems: the moods of children with Prader–Willi syndrome can be very unpredictable. At one moment they can be "all sweetness and light," but within a few seconds, they can deteriorate into an angry outburst. These violent temper tantrums can be triggered by the constraints necessary to curb appetite—food is of great importance to the child with Prader–Willi syndrome. If at all possible, confrontational situations should be avoided, as it can be all too easy to give into requests for extra food under these circumstances. Patterns of bad behavior can become an established routine, leading to yet more dangerous weight gain in the young person with Prader–Willi syndrome.

Testosterone may be helpful in increasing the size of the penis and scrotum. This treatment does not improve fertility, but it can have a beneficial effect on behavioral problems, as the boy will not be so aware of his physical differences from his peers.

THE FUTURE

Insulin-dependent diabetes is one of the more serious problems that may occur during the adult years. The incidence of this disease is higher in persons with Prader–Willi syndrome than in the general population. Regular checks on blood/urine glucose levels should be done, and any symptoms of excessive thirst, frequent passage of urine, or untoward loss of weight must be investigated urgently.

Problems of **obesity** are high on the list of risk factors. Intercurrent respiratory infections can be dangerous for a very overweight child with Prader–Willi syndrome.

A fully independent life is not usually possible for individuals with Prader–Willi syndrome, but work in a sheltered environment can be undertaken.

SELF-HELP GROUP

Prader–Willi Syndrome Association
National Headquarters
5700 Midnight Pass Road, Suite 6
Sarasota, FL 34242
941-312-0400
http://www.pwsausa.org
email: PWSAUSA@aol.com

Retinitis Pigmentosa

ALTERNATIVE NAMES

Rod-cone dystrophy; pigmentary retinal degeneration.

INCIDENCE

There is a group of conditions classified under the name of retinitis pigmentosa. The conditions all have a similar pathology in the retina—the light-sensitive layer at the back of the eye. Modes of inheritance, severity, and the age of onset of symptoms are the distinguishing factors between the different types.

Retinitis pigmentosa is also a feature of some other syndromes: for example, children with one of the mucopolysaccharide diseases (e.g., Hunter syndrome) or with Usher syndrome can have retinitis pigmentosa, among other problems. Between 1 in every 2,000 and 1 in every 7,000 persons is thought to be affected. Many of these people will have only minor visual problems, such as poor night vision.

Both boys and girls can be affected, but the X-linked form of retinitis pigmentosa only affects boys. Prenatal diagnosis is not routinely available at present.

CAUSATION

There appear to be three distinct modes of inheritance of retinitis pigmentosa. Autosomal recessive, autosomal dominant, and an X-linked recessive form have all been described. Around half the persons with retinitis pigmentosa are the sole members of their families with the condition.

The autosomal recessive type appears to be the most common. This type first gives rise to symptoms during the first 20 years of life and progresses until the 50s or 60s, when there is often severe visual loss.

The autosomal dominant type can appear early in the teenage years, but it more frequently begins to give problems later in life, around 40 to 50 years of age. Progress is slower in this type.

The X-linked form is the least common and, of course, only affects boys. This type is frequently the most severe, causing severe visual disability by middle age.

These different types are thought to arise from different gene defects.

CHARACTERISTICS

The basic abnormality in retinitis pigmentosa is a relative decrease in the number of "rods" and "cones" in the retina. These rods and cones are the light receptors and are a vital stage in the process of normal vision. In addition, clumps of pigmented tissue can be seen in the retina. The tiny blood vessels of the retina also show degenerative changes.

All these changes add up, from a clinical point of view, to **reduced vision**. The amount by which vision is reduced is very variable, and some people will manage quite adequately, with only reduced night, and peripheral, vision. The first hint that a child may have retinitis pigmentosa is often a complaint that he/she cannot see as well in the dark as his/her playmates. A further sign is a narrowing of the amount that can be seen peripherally. (People with normal vision probably do not realize just how much they rely on their peripheral vision to make sense of the world around them. It is not until this capacity is lost, and virtual "tunnel" vision becomes the result, that its importance is obvious.) **Color vision** is, at times, also affected.

Retinitis pigmentosa is not associated with other abnormalities elsewhere in the body, except when retinitis pigmentosa is part of other syndromes, such as Usher syndrome or one of the mucopolysaccharide syndromes.

MANAGEMENT IMPLICATIONS

Young children will not show any effects of retinitis pigmentosa if they have the condition. Around 10 to 12 years of age, their vision will deteriorate. Complaints of being unable to see clearly the television or the blackboard at school may be the first intimation that the child has a pigmented retina. An ophthalmologist can confirm the diagnosis by visualizing the retina with an ophthalmoscope.

Comprehensive vision testing is necessary to see if there is any degree of near sightedness. This condition, and any other refractive errors, can be corrected by appropriate lenses, but no glasses can help the basic problem in the retina.

Regular tests of vision throughout life are necessary to determine the rate of progress of the condition. In many cases, progress is slow and only in advanced years is blindness the result. A few children, however, may need special schooling facilities because of their poor vision.

There are night-vision aids available that can help with this aspect of retinitis pigmentosa.

In the USA, trials with vitamin supplements have been undertaken. There has been some suggestion that this treatment may slow the progression of the disease, but no conclusive proof has, as yet, been demonstrated.

THE FUTURE

Careers that rely heavily on excellent vision, such as piloting airplanes, will not be possible for young people with retinitis pigmentosa, but most other careers will be open to affected persons, unless they suffer from the severe and rapidly progressive form. Life expectancy is normal for the person with retinitis pigmentosa. It is only when the condition is associated with some other, more serious, condition (as found in other syndromes), that life expectancy is shortened.

SELF-HELP GROUP

Foundation Fighting Blindness
Executive Plaza I, Suite 800
11350 McCormick Road
Hunt Valley, MD 21031-1014
888-683-5551 or 410-785-1414

Rett Syndrome

INCIDENCE

Rett syndrome has been estimated to occur in approximately 1 in every 10,000 to 12,000 female births, but recent research has shown that the condition is probably more common than was hitherto thought. It is now considered to be one of the more common causes of retardation in girls. The condition seems to affect only girls, there having been no confirmed male cases.

There have been, so far, no biochemical or physiological abnormalities detected during life. Diagnosis is therefore entirely clinical. Definitive criteria have been established internationally.

HISTORY

The syndrome was first described by Dr. Andreas Rett from Vienna in 1966. A number of centers throughout the world that are now collaborating on research into this syndrome.

CAUSATION

At present the mode of inheritance is uncertain, but, as girls only are affected, it would appear that there may be mutation of a gene on the X chromosome. The present hypothesis is that this abnormality is incompatible with life in the male embryo.

From postmortem studies, the brain appears to be surprisingly normal, with no degenerative or storage disease apparent. However, there is suspicion that certain areas in the cortex and basal ganglia may be affected. Evidence suggests that Rett syndrome is a primary genetic disorder that only comes to light as development proceeds. This hypothesis fits the clinical picture. Some defect in the metabolism of epinephrine and dopamine may cause this syndrome.

CHARACTERISTICS

Following a normal pregnancy and birth, the baby develops within the accepted range of normal until around 9 to 12 months, when development ceases. At this stage, the baby may be floppy and placid and show jerky movements. A period of regression then sets in, with loss of the skills already learned. This stage may only last for weeks, but it can persist for many months.

Speech: single words are usually developed, although it is rare for two or more words to be put together. During the regressive stage, these skills disappear.

Physical motor skills of both large and fine movements will be progressively lost. Walking becomes stiff and clumsy. Children previously able to feed themselves will lose this skill. In addition to this loss of voluntary movement, involuntary hand movements such as frequent clapping, wringing, and squeezing are very characteristic of Rett syndrome.

Later, there is a tendency for **muscle wasting** to occur. Deformities of the spine and lower limbs can develop, along with increased muscle tone. Some girls become wheelchair-bound, but many women and girls can walk independently. Scoliosis can be made worse as a result of hypotonia and a sedentary life style.

These facts point to some disturbance in the central organization of movement in the brain.

Breathing: in many girls, the breathing pattern is disturbed, with hyperventilation alternating with periods of breath-holding. During these periods of disturbed breathing, the involuntary movements of the hands increase.

Epilepsy may also occur. Abnormalities are seen on the EEG tracing, and they are particularly evident in young girls when breathing is normal. This unusual finding is characteristic of Rett syndrome.

Learning disability is profound, but it stabilizes around five years of age. Speech is usually completely lost, but eye contact and nonverbal communication can improve after the initial loss. Many girls will be able to assist with their dressing and toilet needs.

Mood swings are common during the regression stage, but they usually decrease with age. Later, many types of moods, such as frustration, anger, or pleasure, occur in response to normal everyday stimuli. At these times, the repetitive hand movements and irregular breathing increase.

MANAGEMENT IMPLICATIONS

Epilepsy: various drugs may have to be tried to control seizures if they are troublesome. Several different drugs or a combination of drugs may need to be given before a suitable drug regimen is found. Changes in the drug therapy may also be needed over time.

Mental handicap: children with Rett syndrome will need assessment and subsequent admittance to schools for children with severe learning difficulties. Reassessment must be carried out on a regular basis to ensure that new needs can be met. Positive therapy in the form of structured training in life skills must be undertaken to prevent further deterioration.

Relative immobility can sometimes lead to **contractures** in joints. Physical therapy is useful in the prevention of this problem. Hydrotherapy is valuable, and children enjoy this form of treatment.

All methods of **communication** should be tried. After 10 years of age some children's communication skills can improve. Thus, it is important that all possible channels of communication are kept open. It must be remembered that although sight and hearing appear to be normal in the girl with Rett syndrome, reaction times are slow. Therefore, patience, understanding, and a quiet environment are necessary to enable maximum benefit from skills training.

Music therapy has been found to be successful in controlling some of the extraneous movements of the hands. Dr. Rett has worked extensively with children in this area of therapy.

THE FUTURE

Children with Rett syndrome commonly survive into their early forties. Occasionally, deaths occur suddenly and unexpectedly in mid-childhood.

An independent life is never possible for sufferers from Rett syndrome, but with careful supervision and behavioral training, a reasonable lifestyle can be attained.

Families will need constant advice and support if the child is to stay in her home environment. Rett syndrome is particularly distressing because early development is normal. Special daycare centers may be able to do much to support families.

SELF-HELP GROUP

International Rett Syndrome Association
9121 Piscataway Road
Clinton, MD 20735
800-818-RETT or 301-856-3334
http://www.rettsyndrome.org
email: irsa@rettsyndrome.org

Reye Syndrome

ALTERNATIVE NAMES

Reye fatty liver syndrome; Reye disease.

INCIDENCE

In the early 1970s, there were reports of a specific condition affecting infants and young children who had been sick with a virus. This condition, if the child survived the original serious illness, could result in permanent handicap. Much more has subsequently been learned about the natural history of the disease. The number of children suffering from handicap due to this cause is not accurately known. In recent years, the incidence is thought to be decreasing. Children of any age, from infancy to around 19 years, can be affected. The younger age group have been seen to be more at risk. All races and both sexes can be affected by Reye syndrome.

HISTORY

Reye syndrome was first described by an Australian pathologist, Dr. Douglas Reye.

CAUSATION

Reye syndrome follows an acute viral infection, such as an upper respiratory tract infection, chickenpox, flu, or a diarrheal illness. Various viruses have been implicated in these forerunning infections.

The use of aspirin to control fever and pain in young children with an infection has been suggested to be an added causative factor in Reye syndrome. About 60% of children with Reye syndrome have taken aspirin before the onset of the acute illness. As a result of this finding, aspirin is no longer prescribed for the relief of pain and fever in children under 12 years of age.

Recent research has suggested that some children who develop Reye syndrome have an underlying genetically determined metabolic defect that predisposes them to the symptoms seen in Reye syndrome following an acute infection.

CHARACTERISTICS

The **acute illness** is one in which persistent vomiting and seizures follow an everyday, often mild, infection. The child becomes irritable and may be aggressive. He/she is confused and lacking in energy. Eventually, drowsiness can lead to delirium and coma, with a potentially fatal outcome. Bleeding from the stomach can follow the persistent vomiting. Abnormal fatty deposits are found in the liver, along with encephalopathy (changes in the brain as a result of the illness) at postmortem.

The diagnosis can be difficult, as Reye syndrome can closely mimic, for example, encephalitis, meningitis, or acute poisoning. The child with any of these serious infections will, of course, need hospital treatment. Liver function and blood clotting tests are necessary to confirm the clinical diagnosis.

The **chronic phase:** if the child survives the acute illness, recovery can be complete with no remaining permanent disability. However, some children will unfortunately be left with a degree of brain damage. This damage may be only slight, but severe mental handicap can occur. If the infection affects babies under one year of age, there is more likelihood of residual disability than if this syndrome affects children over that age.

MANAGEMENT IMPLICATIONS

Acute phase: urgent emergency treatment is necessary to reduce the risk of permanent brain damage. Early intensive treatment has been shown to increase the chance of survival, and also to decrease the risk of permanent brain damage. Intensive care facilities in a hospital are frequently necessary in this acute phase.

Chronic phase: the acute stage of Reye syndrome is a serious illness. The young sufferer will require several weeks of convalescence before he/she is fully well again. Adequate rest, with a nourishing diet and graded physical activity, will be needed. Many children will recover completely from their acute infection and suffer no long-term after effects, but some children will regrettably be left with permanent residual damage. The degree of mental handicap will vary, but it will be severe in some cases. If there is any doubt at all regarding possible brain damage resulting from the original illness, multidisciplinary assessment will be needed. From the results of such assessment, any specific disability is unearthed, and appropriate help can be given. The most severely affected children will need special educational facilities. Careful developmental follow-up over the succeeding years will be necessary. Any problem with movement, speech, or cognitive function will benefit from specialized help from therapists. It is difficult to be more specific, as the after-effects of this illness are so variable.

THE FUTURE

The future will depend very much on the severity of the disability once the acute illness is over. Recovery can be complete, with no sequelae. Alternatively, varying degrees of handicap can remain, affecting the remainder of the child's life. If the child is significantly handicapped, sheltered accommodation and work can be necessary after he/she becomes an adult.

SELF-HELP GROUP

National Reye Syndrome Foundation
P.O. Box 829
Bryan, OH 43506-0829
800-233-7393
http://www.bright.net/~Reyessyn

Riley–Day Syndrome

ALTERNATIVE NAME

Dysautonomia.

INCIDENCE

This condition is rare in general populations. Riley–Day syndrome is largely confined to Ashkenazi Jewish families. The incidence in those families is relatively high, the syndrome being found in approximately 1 in every 3,700 births, and approximately 1 person of Ashkenazi descent in every 100 carries the gene. Boys and girls can be affected equally.

Riley–Day syndrome primarily affects the autonomic nervous system, which controls the involuntary actions of the body as well as functions such as blood pressure and temperature. Some voluntary movements, such as speech, swallowing, and other physical movements, can also be affected.

CAUSATION

Riley–Day syndrome is inherited as an autosomal recessive. The incidence is relatively high in the population at special risk, due to the comparatively closed nature of the community, in which intermarriage has been common. There is no prenatal diagnosis possible at present. Genetic counseling is advisable for families who already have a member with the condition.

CHARACTERISTICS

It is only the clumping together of a number of fairly nonspecific symptoms in a child with a family history of the disorder that can lead to suspicions of the presence of Riley–Day syndrome. All children with the syndrome have the following features:

No **tears** are ever shed by a child with Riley–Day syndrome. This absence of tears can lead to ulceration of the cornea. Although there is some minimal tear formation in the tear glands, it is so defective as to leave no tears available to overflow onto the cheeks during everyday upsets.

The **tongue** in the child with Riley–Day syndrome is smooth due to the absence of the papillae that are normally seen.

Other common signs that affect up to 95% of children with Riley–Day syndrome include:

Blotching of the skin, due to the primary disorder in the autonomic system that controls the contraction and dilatation of the blood vessels. This skin condition is particularly noticeable when the child is excited.

Temperature control, also regulated by the autonomic nervous system, is unstable, and can become dangerously high or low. Excessive sweating, in an endeavor to lower a high temperature, is frequently seen in these children.

Pain is not felt as acutely as normal. This condition might seem like an advantage, but pain has the function of giving warning of injury or disease so that action can be taken to avoid further damage. If this built-in warning system does not function adequately, injuries can continue and disease processes can become dangerously advanced before treatment is given. The ability to distinguish between heat and cold is also often diminished—again increasing the risk of injury.

Lack of coordination of limbs when performing everyday activities is noticeable in the child with Riley–Day syndrome. In addition, an unsteady gait is often seen.

Speech can be adversely affected by the relative lack of coordination of the muscles of tongue and throat.

Scoliosis, together with general poor growth, can be a problem.

Intelligence is usually normal in children with Riley–Day syndrome, but emotional instability is common, with wild swings of mood from elation to misery.

Blood pressure control can be unreliable. Hypotension is especially likely to occur when the child gets up from a lying or sitting position. This condition can cause temporary loss of consciousness at times.

Other less common, but nevertheless important, features include **swallowing difficulties** in infancy, which can make feeding a problem in the early days of life. **Uncontrollable vomiting** can also add to the problems of adequate nutrition in this age group. Inhalation pneumonia is an ever-present threat when these two problems are encountered in infancy.

MANAGEMENT IMPLICATIONS

Eyes: extra special care must be taken to protect the eyes of children with Riley–Day syndrome. Dust that would normally be washed away by tears can cause serious abrasions on the cornea, with possible subsequent ulceration. Therefore, any foreign body in the eye must be treated with extreme care. The eye must be adequately cleansed, and the application of a lubricating antibiotic ointment is a necessary precaution.

Infections of any kind must receive adequate and early treatment, due to the instability of temperature control. This lack of control predisposes the child to febrile seizures, so cooling measures must accompany treatment of the underlying cause of the fever.

Pain insensitivity must be mentioned to teachers when schooldays are reached so that watch can be kept for any potentially damaging incidents.

Speech therapy can help uncoordinated muscle function of lips, tongue, and throat.

Behavior modification techniques may be of value in controlling the emotional instability that can be such a destructive part of the behavior pattern of these children. The help of a clinical psychologist can do much to improve life for the child and his/her family.

During anesthesia, care must be taken with drugs that exert an effect on the autonomic nervous system.

THE FUTURE

Children with Riley–Day syndrome often succumb in early childhood to the effects of the swallowing difficulties that are part of the syndrome's pathology, such as inhalation pneumonia. Pneumonia can also recur in early adult life, with similarly fatal results.

Career prospects can be limited by infections, poor vision caused by previous unrecognized corneal abrasions, and also the emotional lability so frequently seen in people with this syndrome.

SELF-HELP GROUP

Dysautonomia Foundation
20 East 46th Street, Room 302
New York, NY 10017
212-949-6644

Rubinstein–Taybi Syndrome

ALTERNATIVE NAME

Broad thumb–great toe syndrome.

INCIDENCE

This syndrome is a rare disorder, the incidence of which was reported to be only 3 affected in 100,000. (This report only related to the Canadian province of Ontario.) It has been estimated that as many as 1 in every 500 people in institutions for the severely mentally handicapped are affected by Rubinstein–Taybi syndrome. This statistic suggests that this syndrome is a significant cause of severe mental retardation. Because of the variability of the characteristics seen in this syndrome, the diagnosis can, at times, be made only tentatively, which adds to the difficulties of assessing the incidence of Rubinstein–Taybi syndrome.

The condition has been reported from many parts of the world, including Japan and Africa as well as in populations of Caucasian origin. Both sexes can be equally affected.

CAUSATION

The inheritance pattern of Rubinstein–Taybi syndrome is uncertain at present, but in a small number of people with the condition, there is a deletion on chromosome 16.

There is no prenatal test available to detect the condition.

CHARACTERISTICS

Developmental delay is apparent in all children with Rubinstein–Taybi syndrome. The delay affects all aspects of mental and physical development. The degree of delay varies from child to child. Along with the mental retardation come varying degrees of language delay, especially with respect to expressive language. Poor concentration is a common feature.

Microcephaly (head circumference at, or below, the lower range of normal) is a characteristic of this syndrome. The head circumference measurement is an excellent indicator of brain growth, so it follows that all children whose head circumference is markedly smaller than the norm will have some degree of mental retardation.

Physical growth in children with this syndrome is retarded. Final height at 18 years of age will only be on the 50th percentile of standard growth charts.

There are a number of unusual **facial features** associated with Rubinstein–Taybi syndrome, which make the children comparatively easy to recognize. Eyes are widely set apart, and eyelids have a characteristic drooping appearance (ptosis). Eyelashes are often beautifully long. Lazy eye is common, as are refractive errors of the eye. The child's nose is an especially obvious feature, being on the large side and convex in a typical Romanesque manner. The mouth is small, typically with a high, arched palate. Teeth are often overcrowded, with an incomplete "bite."

Finger and **toe** features are among the most frequently found characteristics. Both thumbs and (in nearly all cases) both great toes are broad and flattened at the ends. The great toes are also widely separated from the other toes of the foot (cf. Down syndrome). Occasionally, the terminal bones of thumbs and big toes are bifid, this feature adding to the broad, spatulate aspect of those digits. Other fingers can be broader than usual at the ends, and toes can overlap each other.

Other **skeletal problems** can occur. For example, unusual construction of the lower vertebrae gives rise to an awkward gait.

In boys with this syndrome, undescended **testes** are frequently found.

Many children have excess **hair** on their bodies.

There are a number of other abnormalities that can be associated with Rubinstein–Taybi syndrome, including **heart defects, renal problems, seizures,** and **flame-shaped nevi** on foreheads or backs of necks. It is unusual for all these features to be found in one individual, but they occur with sufficient regularity to make remembrance of them necessary when caring for a child with this syndrome.

A **happy personality** is a frequent feature of children with Rubinstein–Taybi syndrome. They are sociable, and possibly a little overfriendly, which makes extra care necessary when the child comes in contact with strangers.

MANAGEMENT IMPLICATIONS

Developmental delay, and all its educational and social effects, must be assessed and regularly monitored by a multidisciplinary team. Particular areas of delay, such as speech (for example), should receive appropriate therapy. Early teaching of self-help skills will assist both the affected child and his/her family to achieve a better quality of life.

Appropriate **schooling,** geared to the child's assessed abilities, will be necessary when school age is reached. A special school or another institution with appropriate facilities will nearly always be necessary for the child with Rubinstein–Taybi syndrome.

Lazy eye and **refractive errors** (be they near- or far-sightedness, with or without astigmatism) must be assessed and treated appropriately. Lazy eye may need surgery to prevent amblyopia. Refractive errors, more common in children with this syndrome than in the general childhood population, will need corrective lenses. Most children with these errors, however mentally handicapped, will willingly wear their glasses. They appreciate the added dimension of clear vision.

Undescended **testes** will need operative procedures to bring these organs down into the correct position in the scrotum. Malignant change or damage due to trauma are both risks if this correction is not made.

Surgery may also be necessary on **toes** if the big toe is so large and displaced as to give rise to difficulties in finding suitable shoes.

Children with Rubinstein–Taybi syndrome can suffer from **urinary tract infections** more frequently than their peers, particularly if there are associated renal abnormalities. These infections must be recognized and treated with the appropriate antibiotic when they occur.

Seizures, if they occur, must be treated with anticonvulsant drugs.

Obesity can be an added problem in the later childhood years. It should receive a dietitian's advice and monitoring.

Teeth, if overcrowding and/or malocclusion are present, should receive dental care.

THE FUTURE

Most children with Rubinstein–Taybi syndrome will never be able to lead a fully independent life due to their mental handicap. Full-time care will be necessary for practically all individuals. Life span is thought to be within the normal range, as long as there are no potentially life-threatening heart or renal abnormalities present.

A specific type of brain tumor is more common in people with this syndrome, and it can have fatal consequences.

SELF-HELP GROUP

Rubinstein–Taybi Parent Group
P.O. Box 146
Smith Center, KS 66967
913-697-2984

Sanfilippo Syndrome

ALTERNATIVE NAME

Mucopolysaccharidosis 3.

INCIDENCE

Sanfilippo syndrome is one of the mucopolysaccharide diseases. The mucopolysaccharides are complex sugars. The defect in Sanfilippo syndrome is a lack, or deficiency of, a specific enzyme that breaks down one of these complex sugars. Due to this defect, there is an accumulation of the particular sugar in the organs and tissues, and this build-up causes the signs and symptoms of the disease. There are at least four subtypes of this syndrome, but they all are similar clinically. The subtypes are known as Sanfilippo A, B, C, and D. The difference in these four types is in the actual enzyme involved. Sanfilippo A is the most common type.

Around 1 in 25,000 live births exhibit this enzyme deficiency. Boys and girls are equally affected.

HISTORY

With advanced biochemical techniques, the specific enzyme defects that occur in all the mucopolysaccharidoses have been found. All of these diseases have a similar clinical picture, which places great emphasis on certain specific signs and symptoms in each syndrome that result from the specific sugar metabolism affected. (See Hunter, Hurler, and Morquio syndromes.)

CAUSATION

Sanfilippo syndrome is inherited as an autosomal recessive genetic defect. Even though the enzyme for each subtype is different, the end result in all types is that excess heparin sulfate is excreted and stored in large amounts in the body due to the deficiency of the specific enzyme.

The condition can be identified prenatally by chorionic villus sampling at around the tenth week of pregnancy.

CHARACTERISTICS

Children with Sanfilippo syndrome are normal babies at birth, and initial developmental milestones are within the normal range. At around two to three years of age, or maybe even later—at early school age—normal developmental progress slows.

Mental and motor development: sadly, after the initially normal growth and development in all areas, there is rapid mental and physical decline between the ages of two and five years. Most intellectual abilities and self-help skills are quickly lost. The child becomes agitated and upset by the smallest changes in routine. Bizarre behavior patterns in the child are also noticed, similar to those seen in severely demented older people. Within a relatively short time, the child is confined to bed by his/her inability to walk or to control his/her movements adequately.

Sleep disturbances can often be a distressing feature of Sanfilippo syndrome. Parents can become quite exhausted by their baby's unusual sleep pattern, which includes frequent waking during the night.

Growth slows at the same time that mental and motor skills are lost. Although the gross short stature of Hunter and Hurler syndromes is not seen, children with Sanfilippo syndrome rarely grow beyond the 25th percentile on standard growth charts.

Facial features: there is a mild coarsening of the features, similar to that seen in the other mucopolysaccharide diseases, although, again, this condition is not as marked as in the other diseases with a similar background. Tongue and lips become enlarged out of proportion with the rest of the face, and head size also increases.

Frequent **upper respiratory tract infections** are another feature of babies with this syndrome. Such infections can, of course, add to the sleeping problems as the baby is distressed by his/her blocked nose and all the other unpleasant symptoms of a head cold.

Deafness is thought to occur later in childhood, due most probably to the frequent upper respiratory tract infections. Hearing can be difficult to check accurately due to the severe mental retardation from which children with Sanfilippo syndrome suffer.

Joints: as in the other mucopolysaccharide diseases, there is some restriction in the movements of the joints, which together with the loss of other motor skills, leads to lack of mobility.

All these signs and symptoms can be directly traced to the accumulation of the specific complex sugar that is continually being laid down in the tissue, and particularly, in the central nervous system in Sanfilippo syndrome.

MANAGEMENT IMPLICATIONS

Once the diagnosis has been made with certainty, parents should be sensitively counseled as to the future. It is incredibly hard to watch your seemingly normal baby deteriorate in all ways so rapidly and completely. Parents will need to be helped through the normal bereavement processes—denial, anger, guilt, and final acceptance, for the loss of a normal child is as truly a bereavement as is death.

Learning difficulties: unusual and unpredictably inappropriate behavior is often the first sign of the regression from continuing normal development. The formerly mild-mannered child will not be amenable to following the normal, well-established routine of the household and will exhibit temper tantrums for no obvious reason. Previously well-known and practiced self-help skills, such as feeding and toilet training, will be lost.

During this stage, patience and understanding are vital, and parents will need to be helped through each problem as it arises. They will also need opportunities to recharge their own batteries and to give a little time to the rest of their family. Schooling for severely handicapped children will eventually be necessary.

Hearing should be assessed, if possible. Testing in itself can prove difficult, and even if it is thought that hearing aids would prove to be beneficial, it is unlikely that the child will tolerate them.

THE FUTURE

The outlook for children with Sanfilippo syndrome is bleak. Death usually occurs before the twentieth birthday is reached, the sufferer being bed-ridden in a severely demented state.

Research is continuing into both enzyme replacement and gene therapy.

SELF-HELP GROUP

National MPS Society
102 Aspen Drive
Downington, PA 19335
610-942-0100
http://mpssociety.org

Shwachman Syndrome

ALTERNATIVE NAMES

ALTERNATIVE NAMES

Shwachman–Diamond syndrome; Shwachman–Bodian syndrome; Burke syndrome.

INCIDENCE

Shwachman syndrome is a rare disorder affecting a number of bodily systems, and it is the second most common cause of disorders of the pancreas. Both boys and girls can be affected. The condition can be diagnosed in the newborn period by certain specific skeletal features. Later in childhood, the other characteristics will become apparent.

At present, there is no prenatal diagnosis possible.

CAUSATION

Shwachman syndrome can be inherited in an autosomal recessive manner, but it can also arise spontaneously.

CHARACTERISTICS

During the early days of life, Shwachman syndrome can be suspected if the baby has **abnormally short ribs,** with other variable bony abnormalities in the chest wall as well.

Later in childhood, the following features will point to the presence of the condition:

The failure of the pancreas to secrete an adequate amount of digestive enzymes will lead to **diarrhea,** with the bowel movements containing much undigested fat that makes them bulky and frothy.

A **vitamin deficiency** of the fat-soluble vitamins (Vitamins A, D, E, and K) will be a further problem associated with the inability of the pancreas to digest food materials.

(Occasionally, the pancreas manages to secrete sufficient enzyme so that the above symptoms do not occur to any great extent. Examination of the enzymes in the duodenum will, however, show that there is some degree of pancreatic insufficiency.)

Growth is affected in practically all children with this syndrome. Growth generally runs along the lower percentiles of standard growth charts, and the child's final stature will be short. Other bones besides those in the chest can be involved and can be responsible for the poor growth.

A mild **developmental delay** is also a relatively common feature, although it is not inevitable.

The **blood** system is affected to differing degrees in children with Shwachman syndrome There is frequently a relative decrease in all the main constituents of the blood. These decreases appear to occur from time to time in a cyclical fashion.

At the times when the blood is especially affected, the condition will lead to the other important characteristic, repeated **infections** of all kinds. These are especially common in young children with Shwachman syndrome, and infections of the respiratory tract are the main type encountered. All types must be treated urgently.

INVESTIGATIONS

Specialized hematological and gastrointestinal techniques are needed to confirm the clinical suspicions that a child may be suffering from Shwachman syndrome.

MANAGEMENT IMPLICATIONS

If diarrhea is troublesome—showing that the pancreas is severely affected—**replacement pancreatic enzymes** will need to be given on a regular basis.

Regular doses of **vitamin supplements** are important to avoid vitamin deficiency conditions.

It is also of vital importance that any—even a seemingly minor—**respiratory or gastric infection** is treated urgently and adequately. Antibiotics will need to be given early for bacterial infections, as the child with Shwachman syndrome has a low level of immunity against such infections. A healthy diet with adequate rest and exercise will help to increase the ability of the child to withstand everyday infections.

Developmental checks are important to determine the level of the child's abilities in all areas, so that strengths can be fostered and weaknesses accommodated.

Anemia and other **blood deficiencies** must be borne in mind as possibilities. A pale, listless child with no energy is a sign that a blood test is necessary. Transfusions to replace blood components will be necessary on some occasions.

Orthopedic advice to prevent further deformity is advisable if there are specific bony abnormalities that become obvious as growth proceeds.

THE FUTURE

The future depends very much on the severity of the condition; some children have few problems. Others will have major difficulties with both gastric problems and repeated serious respiratory infections.

Leukemia is also found more commonly in children with Shwachman syndrome.

SELF-HELP GROUP

Shwachman–Diamond Syndrome International
4118 Quincy Street
Saint Louis, MO 63116
877-SDS-INTL
http://www.xmission.com/~4sskids
email: 4sskids@mvp.net

Sickle Cell Anemia

INCIDENCE

Sickle cell anemia (like thalassemia, another inherited blood condition) is only seen in certain racial groups, including populations around the Mediterranean—areas of Greece, southern Turkey, and Italy. Definitive areas of West Africa and southern India also show a high incidence of this inherited disorder, as do also a high percentage—up to 40% of the population—of African Americans. In this latter group, it is thought that the incidence can be as high as 1 in every 625 births. Both sexes are equally affected.

If the parents are known to be carriers of this condition, prenatal tests can be done on the unborn baby.

HISTORY

It has been found that certain people with sickle cell anemia have some protection against the ravages of a particularly virulent form of malaria—a common condition in many parts of the world from which persons with sickle cell anemia trace their ancestry. (It is a debatable point as to which condition is preferable!)

CAUSATION

Sickle cell anemia is inherited as an autosomal recessive condition.

There is a "carrier" state for sickle cell disease, known as sickle cell trait. While people with this trait do not have any signs and symptoms of the disease, it is important that their medical practitioners are aware of their genetic inheritance. Special care will be needed during anesthesia and certain surgical procedures. Apart from these cautions, these people should be firmly reassured that sickle cell trait will have no effect at all on their daily lives.

The basic problem in this condition is the abnormal structure of the hemoglobin (the oxygen-carrying substance in the red blood cells). The red blood cells themselves are distorted from their normal smooth elliptical shape to an elongate, or "sickle," shaped one. It is this unusual shape that is responsible for some of the symptoms of the disease. The particular type of anemia accounts for the manifestations of the disease.

Hemoglobin is an extremely complicated substance, which may be afflicted with a number of other problems besides the "sickling" of the red blood cells (cf. thalassemia), and it is important that the diagnosis of the exact type of hemoglobinopathy (diseases of abnormal blood production) is made as soon as possible, so that the appropriate treatment and care can be given.

CHARACTERISTICS

The first indications that sickle cell anemia is present can occur when the affected baby is around six months old. At that time, swellings on the short bones of hands and/or feet will be noticed. The baby can also be feverish and irritable. The typical swellings are a direct result of the "clumping" of the abnormal red blood cells in the small blood vessels of the affected area of the body. The growing bone is damaged and responds by an over-growth of new bone. Infection may, or may not, play a part in this early manifestation of sickle cell anemia.

In older children and adults, painful **crises,** usually accompanied by a fever, occur when the distorted red blood cells clump together. Any part of the body can be affected—kidneys, liver, lungs, or brain, for example.

As a result of the clumping together of the red blood cells, the blood supply is reduced to—or cut off altogether from—the affected organ of the body. The symptoms suffered will be related to the organ or tissue involved. For example, renal failure may develop if the blood vessels of the kidney are severely affected. Similarly, paralysis of one side of the body can occur if the blood vessels in the brain are blocked by clumps of abnormally shaped red blood cells.

These crises are frequently precipitated by bouts of infection. It is therefore vitally important that infections in children with sickle cell anemia are treated with a degree of urgency.

Strenuous exercise can also lead to the occurrence of a crisis, when the abnormal red blood cells containing insufficient amounts of oxygen are unable to meet the active body's extra need for this vital gas.

Anesthesia will also need to be given with care to sufferers from sickle cell anemia.

Anemia, which causes the child to be listless, pale, and possibly breathless on any exertion, is a persistent hazard for persons with this condition. Exacerbations in the anemic state occur in episodes that are thought to be related to a specific type of viral infection. Again, the anemia is a direct result of the lack of oxygen-carrying power of the abnormal hemoglobin on the red blood cells.

The **spleen,** tucked away up under the left lower ribs and intimately concerned with red blood cell production and destruction, can also give rise to specific problems. There can be a sudden onset of severe anemia with a greatly enlarged painful spleen. This condition is known as a "sequestration" crisis, and it mainly affects babies and younger children, causing them to collapse and need urgent hospital treatment. Transfusion of blood under these circumstances can be lifesaving.

Children with sickle cell anemia do seem to be especially prone to **osteomyelitis** (an infection in the bones of any part of the body). The reason for this proclivity is unclear, but any pain localized to a particular bone must be fully investigated.

Enuresis (daytime or nighttime wetting) can also be a problem. It can persist into adult life and is due to the inability of the kidneys to concentrate the urine properly. Therefore, large quantities of dilute urine need to be passed from the bladder at frequent intervals.

INVESTIGATIONS

Specialized blood tests on both child and parents will confirm the diagnosis of sickle cell anemia. It is important that sickle cell anemia is differentiated from other somewhat similar conditions, as both treatment and outcome are different.

MANAGEMENT IMPLICATIONS

One of the most important aspects of the care of the child with sickle cell anemia is to **educate** and **alert** the parents to recognize the crises that can occur. It can be all too easy to think that abdominal or chest pain is due to some, relatively trivial, childhood condition, when in reality the child is suffering from a flare-up of the inherited condition. Obviously, if other members of the immediate family also suffer from sickle cell anemia, parents will be more easily able to recognize the symptoms attributable to the disease.

Parents should also be taught to recognize the dangerous crises affecting the spleen. Such crises will cause acute abdominal pain, with the tender spleen being easy to feel in the left upper part of the abdomen. Under these circumstances, the need for urgent medical attention should be impressed on the parents.

Each bout of **infection,** of whatever type, must be treated quickly and adequately in an attempt to avoid a crisis due to sickle cell anemia. In young children, prophylactic treatment with oral penicillin has proved effective in preventing serious infections such as those caused by the pneumococcus bacteria.

If a **crisis** does occur, pain-relieving drugs are necessary, together with plenty of fluids to drink. Many of these events can be successfully managed at home if parents fully understand how important it is that their child should have copious fluids and adequate pain-relieving drugs. When attacks are severe, the individual will need to be hospitalized so intravenous fluids can be given. Specific antibiotics will also be necessary to counteract the infection.

Blood transfusion can be necessary at times to counteract severe anemia.

A particular type of infection with a parvovirus—giving rise to a flu-like illness—can have deleterious effects on the bone marrow. Red blood cell production is reduced by this infection, and severe anemia can be the result.

An adequate, nutritionally sound **diet** during childhood can help to reduce to a minimum the serious manifestations of the disease. It is also important that children with sickle cell anemia should not become exhausted and/or overheated by strenuous physical exercise.

Schooling in mainstream schools is possible as long as the teaching staff understands the need for immediate assessment and treatment if the child should complain of severe pain in any part of the body. The dangers of physical over-exertion should also be stressed under these conditions.

Absences—sometimes frequent—from school can undermine the education of the child with sickle cell anemia. Good liaison between home and school, with work sent home when the child feels well enough to study, can do much to minimize problems of this nature.

Bone marrow transplantation has been carried out in a few children, and it has proved to be successful and curative.

Certain **drugs** have also recently been researched in an effort to reduce adverse symptoms, with some success.

THE FUTURE

It is difficult to predict in any one individual child the outcome of sickle cell anemia. Access to quick medical care is of enormous advantage, for it can allow the sufferer to lead a full and productive life.

Genetic counseling is advisable before pregnancy.

SELF-HELP GROUP

American Sickle Cell Anemia Association
10300 Carnegie Avenue
Cleveland, OH 44106
216-229-8600
email: irabragg@ascaa.org

Silver–Russell Syndrome

ALTERNATIVE NAMES

Russell–Silver syndrome; Silver syndrome; Silver–Russell type dwarfism.

INCIDENCE

The exact incidence of this syndrome is not known, but cases have been reported from many parts of the world. All races and ethnic groups seem to be susceptible, and boys and girls seem to be affected equally. (However, there has been an X-linked type of Silver syndrome described that, due to the mode of inheritance, affects boys only. The characteristics of this type are similar to those found in the other types of Silver–Russell syndrome.)

CAUSATION

The mode of inheritance is, at present, not clear. An autosomal recessive inheritance and a dominant inheritance with incomplete penetrance have each been postulated. Suggestions have been made that placental insufficiency may be a factor in the etiology of this syndrome. This lack of adequate functioning of the placenta may in itself be an inherited characteristic.

CHARACTERISTICS

Short stature: babies with Silver–Russell syndrome are born smaller than normal. Growth throughout childhood usually follows along the normal growth lines, but at, or below, the third percentile on the growth charts. A few children have been reported to show a "catch-up" growth spurt around puberty; in these cases, final adult height more nearly approaches the norm, but such growth spurts are unusual.

Asymmetry is seen, involving either one complete half of the child's body or a particular part (for example, a limb or part of the skull). The degree of asymmetry varies markedly from child to child. Often this aspect of the condition is not noticed at birth or during the early months of life. It is only later, when growth proceeds at a rapid rate, that the unusual development is noticed.

Advanced sexual development, particularly in girls, is a common feature of Silver–Russell syndrome. Breast development, menstruation, and adult distribution of hair can all occur earlier than is usual. These effects go alongside elevated levels of gonadotropins in the blood and urine.

The shape of the **head** is another noticeable characteristic among children with Silver–Russell syndrome. The forehead is wide, and the head tapers down to a thin pointed chin, giving the appearance of a triangular shaped face. One further feature of interest is that the anterior fontanelle tends to close later than is usual.

The **hands** of children with Silver–Russell syndrome frequently have an in-turning little finger (cf. Down syndrome). Toes, too, can show minor abnormalities, such as webbing, particularly between the second and third toes.

Cafe-au-lait spots, similar to those seen in neurofibromatosis, are often seen; they can appear on any part of the body. The spots vary in size from those only the size of a small freckle to pigmented areas more than 30 centimeters in diameter.

Children with this syndrome have often been noticed to **sweat** excessively.

The last three characteristics (in head, fingers, and skin) are all variable manifestations of Silver–Russell syndrome. Short stature, asymmetry of parts of the body, small size at birth, and precocious sexual development are the constant findings. The other added variable factors are, however, helpful in making a diagnosis.

MANAGEMENT IMPLICATIONS

There are two aspects of Silver–Russell syndrome that can call for special help in childhood. **Short stature** and possible asymmetry of the skeleton can cause difficulties during school days. Short stature is not usually so marked that the child will need special equipment, as do children with achondroplasia. The asymmetry of the body, if severe and affecting a major proportion of the body, may need to be corrected with, for example, special shoes to aid normal movement. Physical therapy is valuable in helping the youngster to use the appropriate muscles correctly to balance his/her asymmetry.

Precocious puberty may be upsetting to both child and parents. Sensitive explanation, and practical help in school to deal with the everyday aspects of menstruation, will help girls with the syndrome to come to terms with their early sexual development.

THE FUTURE

The degree of affected movement will depend very much upon the position and severity of the skeletal asymmetry, and career choices may be limited by this aspect of Silver–Russell syndrome. People with this syndrome can expect a normal life span.

SELF-HELP GROUP

Association for Children with Russell–Silver Syndrome
22 Hoyt Street
Madison, NJ 07940
201-377-4531

Sjogren–Larsson Syndrome

INCIDENCE

INCIDENCE

Although this syndrome is very rare, its occurrence has been reported in many countries of the world. Extensive research into this syndrome was done in the 1950s in Sweden. In a particular region of that country, the incidence of the condition, named after the two Swedes who performed the research, was found to be around 8 people in 100,000. Both boys and girls can be affected.

There are a number of other syndromes that cause a skin rash similar to that found in this syndrome, but Sjogren–Larsson syndrome can be diagnosed quite specifically by the associated features.

CAUSATION

This syndrome is inherited as an autosomal recessive characteristic. The abnormal gene responsible has not, as yet, been located. Carriers of the condition can be detected by the deficiency of a substance necessary for complete oxidation of a further chemical necessary for correct metabolism.

There is no prenatal test available.

CHARACTERISTICS

Skin: the most obvious feature of Sjogren–Larsson syndrome is the specific skin abnormality. Soon after birth, the baby's skin becomes reddened. Within a few weeks, this redness becomes a typical fish-scale-like rash (icthyosis). The skin is dry and "scaly" to the touch. Parts of the body that approximate most closely together (for example, armpits, elbow creases, the area around the neck, and the lower part of the abdomen) are the most severely affected. These typical skin lesions will persist throughout life.

A further characteristic of Sjogren–Larsson syndrome is **spasticity.** It is usually confined to the lower part of the body. As a result of this spasticity, around three-quarters of the persons with this syndrome are confined to a wheelchair for most of their lives. Legs are stiff with increased tone in the muscles. An increase in muscle tone is also often seen around the mouth region. This condition can cause difficulties in feeding, particularly in the early days of life, and it can also create problems with the subsequent development of speech.

Mental abilities: almost all sufferers from this syndrome have some degree of mental handicap. Some children are only mildly retarded, having an IQ level of between 70 and 90. (This level is defined as "borderline retardation.") Other children are severely mentally handicapped.

These three features are those that must be demonstrated before a diagnosis of Sjogren–Larsson syndrome is made. As mentioned before, a number of other syndromes have icthyosis as part of their pathology, but only Sjogren–Larsson sufferers have the added characteristics of mental handicap and neurological signs.

Eyes: in around one half of the children with Sjogren–Larsson syndrome, there will be a degeneration of parts of the retina. This problem can occur as early as two years old. If it does occur, vision will be affected to a greater or lesser degree, depending on the severity and location of the retinal degeneration.

MANAGEMENT IMPLICATIONS

Skin: the dry scales of certain areas of the skin seen in this syndrome can be very uncomfortable for the afflicted person, due to the associated dryness. Soap, which has a drying quality, should be avoided when bathing children with this condition. Lactic or glycolic acid can be used to remove the dry scales gently. This procedure will need to be done on a regular, continuing basis. Other emollient creams can also be tried in an effort to reduce the dryness. The help of a dermatologist is valuable. Clothing will need to be carefully chosen so that the dry, scaly skin does not catch on fluffy fabrics. Natural fibers, such as cotton, are probably the most suitable. Children, as they grow older, can become acutely embarrassed by their scaly skin, which is so unlike the smooth skin of their contemporaries. Clothing with long sleeves and high necks will do much to reduce everyday embarrassment. Teachers will need to be informed of the child's skin condition when school days are reached, so that appropriate explanations can be given to the child's classmates.

Spasticity: little can be done to relieve this tragic neurological abnormality. In the early days of life, feeding may need extra care due to the tight muscles of the mouth and throat. Speech, for the same reason, may show articulation difficulties. Speech therapy input from an early age will ensure that speech develops as normally as possible. If the mental handicap is severe, it will, of course, give rise to greater problems in speech—and other—areas of development. Regrettably, children with Sjogren–Larsson syndrome will eventually become wheelchair-bound, due to their neurological abnormalities. Good nursing care will be vital to prevent pressure sores.

Mental handicap: It is of vital importance that routine developmental checks are done for these babies and children on a regular basis. Just because Sjogren–Larsson syndrome has been diagnosed does not necessarily mean that the child will be severely mentally retarded; IQ may border on normal. When school days are reached, it is important that the correct school for the child's abilities is chosen so he/she can reach his/her full intellectual potential.

Vision: visual acuity should be continually checked throughout life. Ophthalmic examination will show if there is any retinal degeneration present. Little can be done to improve impairment to vision from this cause, but with routine checks, other refractive problems of far- or near-sightedness or astigmatism can be corrected by appropriate lenses, thereby reducing the visual disability to a minimum.

THE FUTURE

The future outlook is very dependent upon the severity of the neurological and mental disabilities. Life expectancy can be reduced if either of these two aspects is severe.

SELF-HELP GROUP

F.I.R.S.T.
Foundation for Ichthyosis and Related Skin Types
P.O. Box 669
Ardmore, PA 19003
610-789-3995 or 800-545-3286
http://www.libertynet.org/icthyos
email: Ichthyosis@aol.com

Smith–Lemli–Opitz Syndrome

ALTERNATIVE NAME

RHS syndrome.

INCIDENCE

The incidence of this rare syndrome is estimated to be about 1 in 40,000. It is thought that boys and girls are equally affected. The uncertainty about both the incidence and the ratio of affected males and females is due, in part, to the greater ease with which boys with this syndrome can be identified, the genital abnormalities being more readily seen in boys than in girls.

The only prenatal test possible at present is by ultrasound. By this method, the genital abnormalities can be detected.

Genetic counseling is advisable before parents of a child with Smith–Lemli–Opitz syndrome embark upon a further pregnancy.

HISTORY

The name of syndrome was coined from the surnames of the families with whom Dr. Opitz worked.

CAUSATION

This syndrome is inherited in an autosomal recessive manner.

CHARACTERISTICS

Growth failure: This feature can be noted prenatally as well as after birth. Due to the poor growth, both in weight and height, the baby with this syndrome has a low birth weight.

The continuing failure of the baby to thrive adequately after birth is enhanced by **feeding** difficulties. The baby's muscles are weak and hypotonic; as a result, sucking is poor and milk is frequently regurgitated.

Facial features include a high, narrow forehead with a small head (microcephaly). A short, tip-tilted nose; a cleft palate and an underdeveloped lower jaw are also frequently seen. The latter feature adds to the initial feeding difficulties.

Boys have **genital abnormalities,** including a hypospadias, a small, underdeveloped scrotum, or ambiguous genitalia that make it difficult, at first sight, to determine the sex of the baby.

Hands and **feet** also show abnormalities. Extra fingers are seen in around 30% of babies with Smith–Lemli–Opitz syndrome, and webbing of the toes is seen in about 10% of children.

To a lesser extent, **heart and renal defects** are seen in the most severely affected babies.

Learning difficulties are almost always present and can vary from a moderate to a severe degree.

MANAGEMENT IMPLICATIONS

Skilled **nursing care** is vital in the early days of life in order to overcome the feeding difficulties caused by both the unusual facial features and the general hypotonia of the baby. Weight gain improves once the early months are over and the baby's muscle tone and facial features mature.

The **genital abnormalities** will need assessment and treatment by a surgeon specializing in this field. Surgery must also be done at a later date on boys with a hypospadias.

Similarly, extra **fingers** may need surgery at a later date. The webbed toes do not usually cause problems, but they may require surgery later.

Any **heart and/or renal problems** that come to light over the first few weeks of life will need assessment and appropriate treatment.

Developmental checks will determine the level of the child's abilities over the first few years. Parents will need sensitive counseling regarding the difficulties that their son or daughter will experience as he/she matures.

Suitable **schooling** will need to be investigated and provided. Close liaison between health and education authorities is vital to ensure that the most suitable environment is found for the child with Smith–Lemli–Opitz syndrome.

THE FUTURE

Life expectancy is not good for children with the severe heart or renal abnormalities that can be associated with this condition. An independent life is rarely possible due to the learning disability.

SELF-HELP GROUP

Smith–Lemli–Opitz (RSH) Advocacy and Exchange
32 Ivy Lane
Glen Mills, PA 19342
610-361-9663
http://members.aol.com/slo97/
email: bhook@erols.com

Smith–Magenis Syndrome

ALTERNATIVE NAME

Interstitial deletion of chromosome 17.

INCIDENCE

This syndrome is rare, the exact incidence being unknown. It is thought, however, that the true incidence is higher than is classified. More people with the condition are being identified as chromosomal analysis becomes more widespread.

Smith–Magenis syndrome has been represented in all parts of the world. There would seem to be a higher incidence of the condition in boys than girls, although that has not been definitely reported.

CAUSATION

In all cases of this syndrome when chromosome analysis has been done, a deletion in a particular part of chromosome 17 has been found to be the cause. The chromosomal defect is thought to arise sporadically—there being no definitive form of inheritance.

Prenatal screening can be offered to families with one affected child.

CHARACTERISTICS

There have been some cases of Smith–Magenis syndrome diagnosed within the first few months of life. Many cases are not diagnosed, however, until later in childhood when the typical features and behavior patterns become evident.

The following features give clues as to the diagnosis:

Certain **facial features** are found in most children with this condition. A smaller than usual head circumference, occasionally being microcephalic, is common. The middle part of the rather broad face is flattened, and the nose is small in contrast to the prominent forehead. Ears, too, can be of an unusual shape and set low on the head.

Short stature is usual, with delayed growth occurring in the early years of life. Later in childhood, **excessive weight gain** can be a problem.

(Due to this feature, this syndrome can be confused with Prader–Willi syndrome, where short stature and excessive weight gain are also features. In Smith–Magenis syndrome, however, the insatiable appetite found in children with Prader–Willi syndrome is not seen.)

A high proportion of children (around 80%) will be **hyperactive** and show **self-destructive and aggressive tendencies.** Self-destructive aspects include such worrying activities as the child severely injuring his/her tongue and/or lips by continual chewing. Biting—both oneself and other people—is a particular aspect of this condition. There would seem to be a relative insensitivity to pain, which may partially account for this type of behavior.

General hyperactivity will be accompanied by **sleep disturbances,** which may exhaust the family, while the child never seems to tire.

Developmental delay is a further feature frequently found in children with Smith–Magenis syndrome. Retardation varies from moderate to severe. This feature, when combined with hyperactivity and behavior problems, causes grave difficulties in management.

Speech delay is another common problem. The delay can, of course, be related to the degree of mental retardation, but it also seems to be a feature specifically found in children with this syndrome.

Children with Smith–Magenis syndrome occasionally suffer from **seizures.** Also, **congenital heart defects** are sometimes found, and there seems to be a higher incidence than usual of **middle ear infections** in later childhood.

Diagnosis can be confirmed by **chromosome analysis** on a blood sample.

MANAGEMENT IMPLICATIONS

The most difficult aspect in the care of the child with Smith–Magenis syndrome is the control of the aggressive and self-mutilating **behavior.** Specialized assistance from a clinical psychologist knowledgeable about behavior modification techniques will be of immense help.

Routine **developmental checks** on all aspects of physical and mental development is necessary to determine the level of any retardation that may be present. When the child's abilities are known and school days approach, close liaison between educational and health authorities is vital to determine the best education provision for the individual child.

Repeated **ear infections,** if they occur, must be treated quickly and adequately. Checks on hearing should also be done after each attack of severe otitis. The child with this unpleasant syndrome can do without deafness to compound the problems.

Speech therapy can be helpful, but the degree of mental retardation must be borne in mind by therapists when treating these children.

A dietitian's advice on **weight control** can also be valuable to avoid the potential long-term problems—and short-term discomfort—of obesity.

Genetic counseling, with prenatal screening, if there has already been one affected child in the family is necessary before parents pursue another pregnancy.

THE FUTURE

Full-time care will be necessary for those children and adults with the most severe retardation and difficult behavior patterns.

Life expectancy does not appear to be reduced—one patient lived 65 years!

SELF-HELP GROUP

PRISMS
(Parents and Researchers Interested in Smith–Magenis Syndrome)
11875 Fawn Ridge Lane
Reston, VA 22094
703-709-0568
http://www.kumc.edu/gec/support/smith-ma.html
email: acmsmith@nhgri.nih.gov

Sotos Syndrome

ALTERNATIVE NAME

Cerebral gigantism.

INCIDENCE

Sotos syndrome is a rare genetic growth disorder, the true incidence of which is not recorded, although 150 cases have been reported since 1964. Boys and girls are equally affected.

HISTORY

Dr. Jaeken in 1972 reviewed 80 children with the collection of characteristics that make up Sotos syndrome.

CAUSATION

Sotos syndrome is thought to be genetically determined. An autosomal dominant pattern is probable, as some families have more than one member with the same condition. Inheritance may also be sporadic due to a new mutation.

The underlying cause is thought to be a nonprogressive abnormality in the hypothalamic region of the brain.

CHARACTERISTICS

Early rapid **growth** is the most obvious and consistent feature of Sotos syndrome. At birth, babies with Sotos syndrome are usually well above the 90th percentile for length. Growth is rapid throughout the first four or five years of life. Following this time, growth slows, but it still persists along the upper ranges of normal. Final adult height is similarly in the upper ranges of normal, with only a very few exceptionally tall adults being recorded.

The **bone age** in children with Sotos syndrome is advanced.

Tooth eruption and development is also advanced, in line with the other bony characteristics.

Facial features: children with Sotos syndrome have large heads with particularly prominent foreheads. Eyes are downward slanting and are set wide apart. The chin is large, and a high arched palate is characteristic.

Limbs: hands and feet are proportionately large. The arm span frequently can be greater than the child's height!

Learning disability: although by no means invariable, between 50% and 80% (according to different authorities) of Sotos syndrome children have some degree of mental retardation. The disability is generally only mild, but some children are severely retarded.

Other more variable characteristics include the following:

Seizures occasionally occur in this syndrome.

Renal tumors (especially Wilm's tumors) have been reported to have a higher incidence than normal in children with Sotos syndrome.

Clumsiness is evident in many children with this syndrome. It may be part of the underlying cause of the condition, but it could be merely due to the rapid growth that occurs during the early years.

MANAGEMENT IMPLICATIONS

Tall stature can cause problems in the preschool years. Children with Sotos syndrome are both larger and stronger than their peers, and have not, as yet, learned how to control their strength and their actions. Therefore, care must be taken to ensure that these children do not intimidate their playmates. Socialization can be especially difficult if there is also a degree of mental retardation. Strict supervision in playground activities and guidance in suitable forms of self-expression will be needed.

Suitable clothing and footwear can sometimes be a problem in the three- to four-year-old child. He/she will require sizes more usually recommended for a ten-year-old.

Similarly, care must be taken not to expect too much, by way of ability or behavior, from a child with Sotos syndrome. His/her size can belie the developmental stage attained.

Mental retardation: care givers should be alerted to the possibility of learning problem associated with Sotos syndrome. Full assessment of a child's abilities in all areas of development will be necessary to determine suitable and appropriate schooling. Some children with Sotos syndrome may need to be part of programs for pupils with moderate learning difficulties, while others manage quite adequately in mainstream educational establishments.

Seizures, although not a common finding in this condition, will need to be investigated in order that appropriate anticonvulsant drugs can be prescribed.

Wilm's tumor: the higher probability that this renal tumor may occur in a child with Sotos syndrome must be remembered. Most frequently, the first sign of the growth is an abdominal swelling with no other symptoms. Occasionally, pain or blood in the urine are associated symptoms. Surgery, followed by chemotherapy and/or radiotherapy, is the necessary treatment.

THE FUTURE

Children with Sotos syndrome have a normal life span with few complications. As mentioned, Wilm's tumors must be remembered during childhood.

During both childhood and adult life, hypo- or hyperthyroidism is a possibility that must not be overlooked. Appropriate treatment for the condition must then be given.

SELF-HELP GROUP

Sotos Syndrome Support Association
Three Danda Square
Wheaton, IL 60187
708-682-8815
email: sssa@well.com

Spinal Muscular Atrophy

Werdnig–Hoffman disease; Wolfhart–Kugelberg–Welander disease.

INCIDENCE

Classification of the varying types of spinal muscular atrophy is some-what confused; there being a number of different types. Werdnig–Hoff-man disease (infantile type or type 1) and Wolfhart–Kugelberg–Welander (juvenile type or type 3) are the two most common types seen in child-hood. (Type 2 is intermediate in severity between types 1 and 3.)

Signs and symptoms of Werdnig–Hoffman disease are seen early in life, while symptoms of Wolfhart–Kugelberg–Welander disease are usu-ally seen only after the age of two years.

Studies of populations in northeast England report the incidence of Werdnig–Hoffman disease is around 1 in every 25,000, with a slightly lower incidence in that region for the juvenile form (Wolfhart–Kugelberg–Welander disease).

There would seem to be a slightly higher incidence of spinal muscu-lar atrophy diseases in boys than in girls. The juvenile form affects boys less severely than it does girls.

Chorionic villus sampling is available for prenatal diagnosis.

CAUSATION

Most cases of spinal muscular atrophy appear to be inherited as an auto-somal recessive characteristic, but some cases of the juvenile type are inherited as an autosomal dominant. The gene has been mapped to chro-mosome 5.

The basic pathology of all types of spinal muscular atrophy is a degeneration (due to an, as yet, unknown cause) of a particular part of the spinal cord (the anterior horn cells). As a result of this degeneration, changes are seen in the muscles controlled by the nerves arising from the affected part of the spinal cord.

CHARACTERISTICS

Werdnig–Hoffman disease

Werdnig–Hoffman, or type 1, disease is the most severe of the 3 types of spinal muscular atrophy. It is often obvious at birth, when the baby will be extremely **floppy.** Before the baby is born, the pregnant woman may observe that the fetus does not seem to move much. If the condition is not immediately obvious at birth, by 3 months of age, the baby will show definite signs of the disease.

A striking feature of the disease is the difference seen in the movements seen below the baby's neck to the expressive, alert movements of the face. The main part of the baby's body will be weak and will eventually become paralyzed.

A further feature is the rapid, fluttery type of movements (fasciculation) seen in some groups of muscles.

Regrettably, this severe type of spinal muscular atrophy is rapidly progressive, causing **paralysis** of all muscles, including those around the chest that are intimately concerned with respiration. Death, due to respiratory failure, usually occurs sometime after 6 months of age and always before the age of 3 years.

Wolfhart–Kugelberg–Welander disease

In this form (type 3), signs and symptoms are not seen until after 2 years of age. They may even first appear as late as the adolescent years. Affected children will be able to learn to walk, although as the disease progresses, they will have a waddling type of gait.

The child with this condition will have difficulty climbing stairs and will also find it hard to get back on his/her feet again after a fall. (cf. Duchenne muscular dystrophy, with which early stages of Wolfhart–Kugelberg–Welander disease can be confused.)

The disease appears to progress in jumps and starts, often with long periods of time when no further problems are encountered.

As the disease progresses to involve the arms and shoulder girdle, a **tremor** often can be noticed when arms are outstretched.

Scoliosis (a sideways twist to the spine) can be a feature.

Intellectual development is normal.

Type 2 spinal muscular atrophy

Type 2 is intermediate in severity between types 1 and 3. The child is able to sit up unsupported, but she/he cannot stand or walk. The **weakness of the muscles** is a very obvious sign, and in this type, there is wasting of the muscles together with a loss of subcutaneous fat, which makes the child thin and underweight.

Scoliosis and rib deformities due to forced inactivity can give rise to respiratory problems. Many children die, due to this cause, before their tenth birthday.

INVESTIGATIONS

Electromyogram will show a definitive pattern of disorganized muscle activity.

Biopsy of muscles will show specific changes in these tissues, which enable a firm diagnosis to be made.

A specific enzyme deficiency has been found in some sufferers from this group of conditions. Therefore, it may be found that this condition is a metabolic one, caused by a deficiency, or absence, of a vital enzyme.

MANAGEMENT IMPLICATIONS

For the baby with Werdnig–Hoffman disease, only routine care and nursing is possible. Extra care must be taken to prevent pressure sores arising from paralyzed limbs.

Parents must receive practical and emotional help with their handicapped baby. The nature of the disease, together with the inevitable outcome, must be sensitively discussed on an ongoing basis. It is difficult indeed for parents to come to terms with the fact that their baby will have only a short life, and there will be many questions to be answered as the weeks pass.

Bereavement counseling is also of importance following the death of the child. Genetic counseling is advisable when a parents of an affected child envisage a further pregnancy.

The child with Wolfhart–Kugelberg–Welander disease will also need much help and routine care as the disease progresses. Routine developmental checks will determine the rate of development of motor skills, such as walking or climbing stairs.

Help with walking, according to the degree of disability, will probably be needed. Physical therapy skills are extremely valuable in this context. Possible bathing and toilet problems may be encountered—for example, it may be necessary to provide downstairs facilities if climbing stairs is a particular problem.

When school days arrive, teachers must be made aware of their pupil's problems. The child will be unable to pursue many physical activities, and the child should be encouraged to take an interest in more sedentary hobbies and possible later career choices.

Special bathroom facilities may need to be made available at school, depending on the degree of the child's disability. Stairs between classrooms can also cause difficulties.

Careers must be carefully chosen, and the child with spinal muscular atrophy will need to be encouraged to take an interest in those aspects of work that can be undertaken within the limits of the disease.

THE FUTURE

Life expectancy for people with Wolfhart–Kugelberg–Welander disease is near normal.

SELF-HELP GROUP

Families of Spinal Muscular Atrophy
P.O. Box 196
Libertyville, IL 60048-0196
800-886-1762
http://www.abacus96.com/fsma/home.htm

Stickler Syndrome

ALTERNATIVE NAME

Hereditary progressive arthro-ophthalmopathy.

INCIDENCE

This syndrome is thought to affect 1 in every 20,000 live births. Both sexes can be affected equally. Prenatal ultrasound can detect the cleft palate that is a feature in some babies with Stickler syndrome.

The condition can be recognized soon after birth if the "Robin anomaly" (see below) is present. A positive family history of the condition can also help in making the diagnosis.

HISTORY

Stickler syndrome has some features similar to those seen in Marfan syndrome—the eye and joint problems being somewhat similar. It has been suggested that Abraham Lincoln and his son Todd were both affected by Stickler syndrome, although some historical records show that the Lincolns had features more like those associated with Marfan syndrome.

CAUSATION

Stickler syndrome is inherited in an autosomal dominant manner. The affected gene has been mapped to chromosome 12. Not every baby/adult with this syndrome will necessarily show all the features of the condition to the same extent; the expression of the gene being very variable.

CHARACTERISTICS

Eyes: One of the most constant features of Stickler syndrome is myopia (near-sightedness), which can be severe from an early age. As is the case for all myopic people (from whatever cause), retinal detachment is an ever-present risk. Up to half of all children with this syndrome will have a complete retinal detachment at some time during their lives, usually during the first two decades of life. (A retinal detachment occurs when the retina peels off from the underlying structures. Unless swift diagnosis and treatment is undertaken, the result will be permanent blindness.) Marfan syndrome also has myopia as a characteristic, and retinal detachment can also occur as a result of that condition. The dislocation of the lens of the eye seen in Marfan syndrome is, however, not a feature of Stickler syndrome.

Early cataract formation can occur as part of Stickler syndrome, together with possible glaucoma.

Children with Stickler syndrome can have **hypermobile joints** (cf. Marfan syndrome), but more frequently, joints become stiff and at times reddened and enlarged. The joints most commonly affected are ankles, knees, and wrists. The joint features may occasionally be recognizable at birth. Due to the possible swelling of the joints, locking can be a problem following physical exercise.

Stature: Some children with Stickler syndrome can be tall and thin. Others, however, can be of a normal height and of rather a stocky build.

Facial features can be unusual in some children with this syndrome. The bridge of the nose can be flattened, this feature being more frequently found in children with short stature. In conjunction with the flattened features of the mid-face, a cleft palate can also be present. The lower jaw can be small, giving rise to feeding and breathing difficulties in the early days of life (cf. Pierre–Robin syndrome). These two latter features are frequently referred to as the **"Robin anomaly."**

A sensorineural **hearing loss** occurs with a greater frequency than normal.

MANAGEMENT IMPLICATIONS

In the early days of life, the underdeveloped lower jaw can present **feeding difficulties.** Feeding the baby in the upright position may be the only adjustment that is necessary. **Breathing** can also be obstructed by the baby's tongue falling into the back of the throat due to the smallness of the lower jaw. These babies should lay on their sides in a semi-prone position so that the tongue falls forward, away from the throat. Ready access to intubation facilities will be necessary if the Robin anomaly is severe.

Surgical repair of the **cleft palate** will need to be done in the early months of life.

The most important feature to be monitored throughout life is the **visual problem.** Myopia must be assessed and corrected with glasses. Loss, or blurring, of vision must also be urgently investigated to ensure that retinal detachment is diagnosed at an early stage. With early adequate treatment, vision can be saved.

Glaucoma must also be diagnosed and treated in order to preserve vision. (Signs and symptoms of glaucoma include pain in the affected eye, blurring of vision, and complaints of seeing "green haloes" around light sources.)

Eyes will need to be routinely checked for possible cataracts, and appropriate action must be taken where necessary.

The possible hypermobility of **joints** and periods of reddening and swelling means that children with Stickler syndrome should avoid vigorous physical activities. Contact sports of all kinds, in particular, should not be allowed. Episodes of painful red and swollen joints will need appropriate periods of rest and pain relief. The help of a physical therapist is valuable following these episodes.

Schooling will depend on the degree of visual problems present. Special facilities will be necessary for those children with the most severe visual or hearing loss. Careers that depend on good vision or hearing are not suitable.

Children with Stickler syndrome have no loss of intellectual ability.

THE FUTURE

Severe visual loss is the most serious and disabling of the possibilities that can occur with this syndrome. It is thought that all children will have some definite visual abnormalities by the age of 10 years.

With care and gentle graded exercises, joint mobility can be maintained throughout life, although osteoarthritis can develop later in life.

Severe deafness may become an added burden later.

SELF-HELP GROUP

Stickler Involved People
15 Angelina
Augusta, KS 67010
316-775-2993
http://www.stickler.org
email: Houch@southwind.net

Sturge–Weber Syndrome

INCIDENCE

The number of people with this unusual syndrome is unknown, but it is thought to be a rare condition. Both sexes are affected equally.

CAUSATION

The reasons behind the occurrence of Sturge–Weber syndrome are unknown. There does not seem, at present, to be any evidence that it is an inherited disorder. The most probable cause is a new mutation occurring sporadically.

There is no prenatal diagnosis available, but the typical signs on the baby's face are obvious at birth.

CHARACTERISTICS

A **"port-wine" stain** on one half of the baby's face is the most noticeable characteristic seen at birth. This specialized type of "birthmark" follows the course of the fifth cranial nerve. This particular nerve is divided into three branches, supplying the forehead, cheek region, and lower jaw, respectively. The upper branch is most often affected in Sturge–Weber syndrome, but all three branches can be affected, so that the whole side of the face is covered by the purplish mark. The basic cause of this coloration lies in an abnormality in the walls of the tiny blood vessels supplying the skin.

Parts of the blood supply to the **brain** may be affected. On X-ray, specific areas of calcification appear when the child is over the age of two years.

Seizures are often a complication of this syndrome. The usual age of onset is after one to two years old, around the same time that the brain appears altered in X-rays.

Paralysis of one half of the body sometimes occurs.

Both of these latter characteristics are due to the same basic abnormality in the walls of the blood vessels that causes the nevus on the baby's face.

Eyes: glaucoma can at times occur in the eye on the same side as the port-wine stain. The narrow passage that allows the fluid inside the eye to drain becomes blocked by the blood vessel abnormality, causing tension inside the eyeball to increase dangerously. This condition, if not treated, can lead to blindness in the affected eye. The color of the eyes may occasionally differ from each other. The eye on the affected side can be blue, even though the other eye is brown. This characteristic is due to the abnormality affecting the blood vessels at the back of the eye.

MANAGEMENT IMPLICATIONS

"Port-wine" stain: There is no easy treatment for this type of birthmark, particularly if it occupies an extensive area. Laser treatment is available in some centers, but this procedure is time-consuming, as only small areas can be treated at any one time, and expensive. Effective cosmetic cover-up creams are available, but they are more likely to be used later in life rather than in childhood.

Seizures will need to be treated with anticonvulsant drugs, and several drugs or drug combinations may need to be tried before an effective regimen is found. If the seizures cannot be controlled by medication, surgery to specific affected areas of the brain can be of value.

Glaucoma (symptoms of which are pain in the affected eye, blurred vision, and possibly the seeing of green "haloes" around sources of light) needs urgent treatment by eye drops or surgery. Without treatment, blindness can result.

Emotional problems can occur, especially in the teenage years, and also particularly in girls. Teasing about the facial disfigurement can lead children to become withdrawn. The help of a clinical psychologist will be helpful in the most severely affected children.

THE FUTURE

The future will very much depend on the extent, and sites, of the abnormalities in the walls of the blood vessels. If only the skin of the face is involved, there is no threat to life or health. But if the disease is more extensive and affects other blood vessels in the brain, seizures can be a grave problem with potentially fatal results.

SELF-HELP GROUP

Sturge–Weber Foundation
P.O. Box 418
Mount Freedom, NJ 07970
800-627-5482 or 973-895-4445
http://www.sturge-weber.com
email: swf@sturge-weber.com

TAR Syndrome

ALTERNATIVE NAME

Absent radius-thrombocytopenia.

INCIDENCE

TAR syndrome is a relatively rare syndrome, but more than 100 cases have been reported in the literature. There appears to be no special geographical location or ethnic groups in which there are a greater number of cases.

There would appear to be more girls affected than boys. The reason for this finding is thought to be that many males are so severely affected by the condition that death occurs *in utero*.

Ultrasound examination during pregnancy—from 18 weeks onward—can detect the specific abnormality in the baby's arms.

HISTORY

The common name of this syndrome is an acronym of the abnormalities found—*t*hrombocytopenia, *a*bsent *r*adius.

CAUSATION

This syndrome is inherited in an autosomal recessive manner.

CHARACTERISTICS

Blood system

Thrombocytopenia—a reduction in the number of platelets circulating in the blood—is one of the main features of this syndrome. (Platelets play a vital role in the normal clotting of blood.) In the most severe cases, there are also abnormalities in the function of the platelets that are present.

Thrombocytopenia will result in abnormal **bleeding** in various parts of the body—for example, bleeding from the bowel, nose bleeds, and excessive bruising from very minor injuries.

More than 90% of new born babies with this condition will suffer from some episode of bleeding during their first few months of life. This bleeding can be severe and life-threatening, and it is thought that around 30% of babies with this syndrome die before one year of age due to uncontrollable bleeding.

If the first few critical months are survived, the episodes of bleeding tend to occur in a more episodic fashion, with incidents related to some form of bodily stress, such as an infection or a necessary surgical operation. Even in the most severely affected baby, the platelet count will tend to improve as the years go by—so that, even in these cases, the episodes of severe bleeding will tend to occur only with stressful life events.

Anemia can be an ever-present concern, due to the blood loss through the frequent bleeding episodes as well as other possible blood abnormalities.

Skeletal system

The other main feature of TAR syndrome is the absence of the **radius** from the child's forearm. (The radius is one of the two long bones linking the elbow to the wrist.) Both arms are usually affected by this abnormality.

In some children, there are abnormalities of the bones of the **hands.** In addition to this possible bone abnormality, further deformities can occur in the hands due to the unequal and unusual pull of the muscles that normally act on the radius, but which now act on the bones of the wrist. Children with this deformity will—understandably—be slower than their peers in gaining manual dexterity. However, motor function is eventually developed, with help and practice.

Other problems can occur in different parts of the skeleton. For example, **hips** can be dislocated; **knees** can be stiff from the occasional dislocation of the knee cap; or **ribs** and **spine** can show abnormalities. These latter effects can cause the child to have a **short stature.**

These latter skeletal features will vary from individual child to individual child.

The blood and skeletal characteristics described above are always found in children with TAR syndrome, but the following features can also occur:

- **Heart defects** of various types can be present. Tetralogy of Fallot (in which there are 4 specific heart abnormalities) or an atrial septal defect (or a "hole" between the two upper chambers of the heart) are the most commonly found problems.

- **Mental retardation** can very occasionally occur if there has been bleeding into the brain at an early stage in life.
- **Allergy** to cow's milk has been reported in an above average number of children with TAR syndrome.

MANAGEMENT IMPLICATIONS

Blood: Each episode of bleeding must be treated with urgency. This approach is especially important in the early days of life when these events are more common. Transfusion of either whole blood or platelets may be necessary when bleeding is severe.

As the baby matures and begins to crawl and walk, the inevitable **minor injuries** must be reduced to a minimum. Again, urgent medical treatment must be sought if serious bleeding occurs.

It is also important to avoid **infections** as far as is possible without overprotecting the child. Each bout of infection should be treated aggressively so as to reduce the risk of bleeding due to the abnormal clotting mechanism found in TAR syndrome.

Anemia should be checked for whenever a child appears listless, lacks energy, or looks especially pale. Such checks will, of course, be particularly important after an episode of bleeding.

Skeletal: The advice of an orthopedic surgeon can be necessary. Possible realigning of muscles in the arm to improve function may be necessary.

Physical therapy help, in the early days, when hand and arm dexterity are being learned, is valuable.

Orthopedic appliances, in the form of braces, can be helpful, and should be fitted early for maximum effect.

Possible **heart defects** will need to be assessed and treatment decided upon by a pediatric cardiologist.

Schooling will need to be geared to the child's individual physical abilities. (Intellectual ability is generally normal, unless intracranial hemorrhage in the very early days of life has left irreparable brain damage.) Children with TAR syndrome will need extra help with writing and drawing skills. Typewriters and/or word-processors can be an option at a later date.

Contact sports should be avoided, due to the ever-present possibility of bleeding from even minor trauma.

Careers will need careful consideration, given the physical and bleeding problems.

Any **cow's milk allergy** will need dietary advice, and an alternative milk supply—goat's milk or soy milk—must be provided.

THE FUTURE

Outlook for life expectancy is good once the difficult, and potentially fatal, days of early childhood are successfully passed.

Women will tend to suffer from heavy menstrual periods, and they must watch for anemia.

SELF-HELP GROUP

T.A.R.S.A. –Thrombocytopenia Absent Radius Syndrome Association
212 Sherwood Drive
Egg Harbor Township, NJ 08234-7658
609-927-0418
email: purinton@earthlink.net

Tay–Sachs Disease

ALTERNATIVE NAME

GM2 gangliosidosis.

INCIDENCE

This condition is usually seen only in Ashkenazi Jewish families, where the incidence is thought to be as high as around 1 in every 4,000 live births. A further population group in which this serious condition occurs is French Canadians. Older children and adults are virtually never seen with Tay–Sachs disease, as death inevitably occurs in early childhood.

Boys and girls can be equally affected.

CAUSATION

Tay–Sachs disease is inherited as an autosomal recessive. There are large numbers of people in the particular population groups mentioned above that carry the abnormal gene; the number of carriers is thought to be as high as 1 in every 25 people. Therefore, in spite of the early deaths of persons with the disease, there is still a great reservoir of people carrying the genetic source of this serious condition.

Tay–Sachs disease is an example of a condition that arises because of a specific enzyme defect. This deficiency allows certain chemical substances to build up in various parts of the body. The chemical excesses then given rise to the specific characteristics of the disease. The enzyme involved in this case is hexosaminidase A. The substance that is not adequately metabolized, due to the lack of this enzyme, is a ganglioside.

Prenatal diagnosis is available by chorionic villus sampling.

CHARACTERISTICS

Tay–Sachs disease can be divided into two types, which are distinguished by the times when the typical signs and symptoms make their appearance. In the "infantile" type, the characteristic features begin to appear within the first six months of life. Typical features of the "late infantile" type (also known as Sandhoff disease) will not show until the child is around two to three years old. In this latter type, two enzymes are involved—hexosaminidase A and B. In both types, the features are the same; only the timing is different. All features are due to an abnormal storage in various parts of the body, particularly in the gray matter of the brain, of the GM2 ganglioside.

Vision: In the infantile type of Tay–Sachs disease, the baby of around six months of age will begin to disregard the kinds of movements around her or him that had previously attracted her or his attention. On ophthalmic examination, there will be seen a cherry red spot on a particular part of the retina, which results directly from the build-up of ganglioside in this part of the eye. Within a very short time, the baby's vision will deteriorate so much that she or he will be quite blind, usually by one year of age.

An **increased "startle" response** will be seen—for example, a person who has been nearby for some time will suddenly make the baby jump. Part of the reason for this increased "startle" reaction may be, in addition to failing vision, a **hypersensitivity to sound.** This feature is one of the earliest signs that the disease may be present.

Loss of skills already learned is an early sign of Tay–Sachs disease. The baby who will have been gurgling, smiling, lifting his/her head, and vigorously moving his/her arms and legs will become limp and unresponsive. This developmental regression can be devastating to the parents who have been watching with delight their baby's increasing awareness of his/her surroundings. As with all the metabolic conditions, the deterioration of a seemingly normal baby can be almost unbelievable.

Seizures commonly begin to occur during the second year of life. Often, they will take the form of outbursts of inappropriate laughter. The EEG will show abnormalities in association with this event. These seizures can be very difficult to regulate, and a number of anticonvulsant drugs may need to be tried before some degree of control is gained. As the disease progresses, the episodes of seizures tend to lessen spontaneously.

Hypotonia, or a generalized weakness of all the muscles, rapidly occurs. The baby who previously had been rolling over and attempting to pull his/her head and shoulders into a sitting position will cease to try this maneuver. He/she will lie apathetically in the crib, becoming more and more unresponsive to his/her surroundings. Only sudden loud noises will cause a "startle" reaction, along with the outbursts of laughter that denote a seizure.

The baby's limbs will eventually become stiff with exaggerated reflexes until a complete spastic paralysis results.

Head size can increase rapidly due to the deposition of abnormal material in the brain. This condition can give the appearance of hydrocephalus, although that is not the true cause of the increase in head circumference. (Hydrocephalus implies an increase in size of the ventricles in the brain containing cerebrospinal fluid.)

The final outcome of this tragic disease is death by the age of three to four years. In the late infantile type (Sandhoff disease), the characteristic features do not begin to make their appearance before two to three years of age, but a rapid deterioration, similar to that seen in the infantile type, proceeds, and death usually occurs between the ages of five and ten years.

MANAGEMENT IMPLICATIONS

Support for, and education of, the parents is a vital part of handling this tragic genetic condition. Parents will need explanations about the inheritance of their baby's illness, the cause of the disease, and the expected age of the final outcome.

Appropriate **nursing care,** together with help for parents with an affected child at home, is virtually all that can be done. Full-time nursing care will eventually be a necessity.

Genetic counseling for couples considering a further pregnancy is advisable so that the risks of having another child with the condition can be estimated.

SELF-HELP GROUP

National Tay–Sachs and Allied Disease Association (NTSAD)
2001 Beacon Street, Suite 204
Brighton, MA 02135
800-906-8723
http://www.ntsad.org/ntsad/contact.htm
email: NTSAD-Boston@worldnet.att.net

Thalassemia

ALTERNATIVE NAMES

Cooley anemia; Mediterranean anemia.

INCIDENCE

Like sickle cell anemia, thalassemia is a hemoglobinopathy. It only occurs in certain racial groups—mainly in tropical and subtropical parts of Europe, Africa, and Asia.

As the alternative name Mediterranean anemia implies, there is a high incidence among people from around the Mediterranean Sea; the disease being virtually unknown among persons of Northern European descent. The incidence is variable, but among some populations, it can be as high as 1 in every 100 births.

Twenty percent of the populations of Turkey and Greece are thought to suffer from the disease. There is also a high incidence in Burma and Thailand.

Both sexes are equally affected.

Prenatal diagnosis by chorionic villus sampling at 10 weeks of pregnancy and/or fetal blood sampling at 20 weeks of pregnancy is possible.

It is important that thalassemia major (which is discussed here) is definitively differentiated from the milder form, thalassemia intermedia, as the course of the diseases and their treatments differ from one another.

HISTORY

The name *thalassemia* was deduced from "thallus," which means an "inland sea," that is, the Mediterranean.

CAUSATION

Thalassemia is inherited as an autosomal recessive condition. The basic abnormality is one of deficient production of hemoglobin—the oxygen-carrying part of the blood found in the red blood cells. One of the specific globulins necessary for the proper metabolism of hemoglobin is not synthesized adequately, and that leads to anemia.

There are two main types of thalassemia—alpha and beta—with a number of complicated variants of both the alpha and beta types. A particularly severe form of alpha thalassemia results in still-birth or death of the affected baby within a few hours of birth.

CHARACTERISTICS (BETA-THALASSEMIA)

The baby with thalassemia is usually healthy at birth, but by 3 to 6 months old she/he will show signs of:

- **anemia:** The baby will become pale and listless, unwilling to take feedings, and he/she may vomit what little food is taken;
- **jaundice** may also be present from an early stage. This yellow coloration of the skin and mucous membranes is caused by the more rapid than usual breakdown of the red blood cells.

Enlargements of the **liver** and **spleen** are also specific features associated with thalassemia.

These characteristics are due to:

- the body attempting to produce red blood cells in parts of the body other than the bone marrow;
- changes relating to the anemia, which by putting an extra load on the heart causes back-pressure on the liver;
- extra deposits of iron-containing substances, which are, in turn, a long-term consequence of the anemia.

Bones can eventually become thinned as a result of the body's attempts to produce adequate hemoglobin for daily needs. This condition can ultimately lead to fractures and deformity.

COMPLICATIONS

The following complications are mainly secondary effects due to the excess storage of iron in the body. They are caused both by the disease itself and by the necessity of frequent blood transfusions.

Heart arrhythmias can be difficult to control and can be fatal.

Cirrhosis of the liver can lead to possible eventual liver failure.

Diabetes can also occur. The disease results from the failure of the specific cells in the pancreas to produce adequate insulin because of the iron overload.

MANAGEMENT IMPLICATIONS

In severe cases of thalassemia, **frequent blood transfusions** are necessary to combat the persistent anemia. Specialized control of the type of blood given and the frequency of the transfusions will be necessary to reduce complications to a minimum.

Removal of the spleen—**splenectomy**—may be necessary. Extra care must be taken following this procedure to protect against infections of all kinds. For example, if a child has a fever for no obvious reason, hospital admission to discover the source of the infection will be urgently needed. Parents must be advised to contact a hematology clinic or their own doctor under these circumstances.

In addition to needing frequent blood transfusions, the affected individual must undergo special chelating (iron-removing) treatment in order to minimize the amount of iron stored in various parts of the body. This treatment can be done either by a subcutaneous infusion with a special "pump," or by giving the substance together with the blood at the time of transfusion. Vitamin C is a necessary dietary additive to assist in the removal of iron. (Given the necessarily long-term nature of this chelating process, which seems to have little obvious effect, parents can at times find it difficult to insist that their child follows these routines. Therefore, explanations and encouragement are a necessary part of the treatment.)

It is important that the development and **growth** of children with thalassemia are regularly checked. Height and weight should be plotted serially on a percentile chart. Also, in children under the age of 12 years, yearly X-rays of the bones of the hand and wrist should be taken to measure bone growth.

Schooling for the child with thalassemia will probably be affected by the frequent absences necessary for transfusion purposes. Liaison between home and school, with work sent home when the child is feeling well enough, will ensure that the child will keep close touch with peers. Teachers should also have a basic understanding of the effects of the disease on their pupils.

Close watch, on a regular basis, will need to be kept for signs of liver, cardiac, and endocrine complications of thalassemia. **Blood tests** to determine liver, pancreatic, and thyroid functions will need to be performed routinely.

Every person suffering from one of the hemoglobinopathies should wear a **medical alert bracelet** so that, in case of emergency, medical staff will be aware of the inherited disease and the need for extra care in treatment.

Emotional and practical support for both parents and child are an important part of care. A balance must be kept to ensure that the need for constant care and treatment does not lead to overprotection. Striking this balance can be an especially difficult problem during adolescence, when the affected child must learn to take control over his/her treatment. A good hematology department can do much to help with this transition into adulthood, as can an appropriate self help group.

THE FUTURE

For people with severe thalassemia, life expectancy is shortened, largely due to the effects of the iron overload in various tissues and organs of the body. With the improved methods of chelation, however, the outlook is improving.

Genetic counseling is advisable for families suffering from this inherited disease.

Bone marrow transplantation—ideally before the age of 12 years when damage by excess iron is less likely—is the treatment currently being explored. Research continues into a chelating agent that can be taken orally.

SELF-HELP GROUP

Cooley's Anemia Foundation
129-09 26th Avenue, #203
Flushing, NY 11354
800-522-7222 or 78-321-2873
http://www.thalassemia.org
email: ncaf@aol.com

Tourette Syndrome

ALTERNATIVE NAMES

Giles de la Tourette syndrome; multiple motor and vocal tics; coprolalia generalized tic.

INCIDENCE

It is thought that this distressing condition may be greatly under-diagnosed due to the considerable degree to which the severity of the disease, the time of onset, and the social disability caused can all vary. Research has put the occurrence of the condition as high as between 1 in 2,000 and 1 in 3,000 for boys, and between 1 in 5,000 and 1 in 10,000 for girls. Thus, boys would appear to be around three times as likely to be affected as girls.

CAUSATION

Tourette syndrome is thought to be inherited as an autosomal dominant condition. However, a high proportion of sufferers have no family history of the syndrome, so other factors may be involved. Birth injury, or the possibility of several genes being involved, are other suggestions as to etiology.

There are no known means of diagnosing Tourette syndrome other than on clinical findings.

CHARACTERISTICS

The age of onset of symptoms varies greatly, ranging from 2 to 21 years. The most frequent age at which problems become obvious is around seven years old.

Tics are of two types:

- **Motor tics**—involuntary movements of face, limbs and body. These unusual movements include eye-blinking, facial grimacing, shrugging of shoulders, and head and arm jerks. For a diagnosis of Tourette syndrome to be made, these, and other, tics must be continually present for over a year. (Many children go through a stage where one or two tics occur, perhaps copied from a friend or even an elderly neighbor, but such gestures are eventually forgotten and are not replaced by other involuntary movements.)

- **Vocal tics**—coughing, sneezing, sucking, throat-clearing, sniffing, and other unusual noises. At times the involuntary shouting of inappropriate words or phrases, including obscenities, can make life extremely difficult for parents and companions of the affected child. The involuntary use of obscene words and phrases (or in some cases, obscene gestures) is found in approximately one-third of all cases of children and/or adults affected by this syndrome. It is a particularly socially disabling facet of the condition, and one that cannot be readily controlled. Vocal tics generally make their appearance some time after the motor tics have become established.

Obsessive behavior is also a common feature of this syndrome. Repetitive actions and patterns of behavior can be another seriously disabling problem.

Reduced attention span can make life difficult.

The whole pattern of Tourette syndrome is fluid, and symptoms may vary in severity from week to week. Some particular problem may disappear for a time, only to reappear again at a later date.

Remissions can occur in some children, but the tics, both motor and vocal, and obsessive behavior will usually reassert themselves again after a brief interval of respite.

MANAGEMENT IMPLICATIONS

Various drugs have been, and are still being, tried to reduce the motor and vocal tics. Results have been variable, but some success has been achieved.

Schooling can be an especially difficult problem, due both to the child's lack of concentration and to the difficult obsessive behavior and repetitive multiple tics. Education in small classes, where a variety of difficult behavior patterns can be contained, may be beneficial. It is of vital importance that the teaching staff is made aware of the diagnosis, so that appropriate care and teaching methods can be employed.

THE FUTURE

Tourette syndrome is not a life threatening disorder, but normal career prospects can be markedly limited by the symptoms. Social contact is also difficult, or even impossible, if the sufferer is severely affected.

SELF-HELP GROUP

Tourette Syndrome Association
42-40 Bell Boulevard
Bayside, NY 11361-2820
718-224-2999
email: tourette@ix.netcom.com

Treacher Collins Syndrome

ALTERNATIVE NAMES

Dysostosis mandibulofacial; Franceschetti–Klein syndrome.

INCIDENCE

The number of people suffering from this particular syndrome is not known. A number of families in which the disease has recurred through-out several generations have been described and studied.

HISTORY

Dr. Treacher Collins first described people with the particular characteristics seen in this syndrome in a paper presented to the Ophthalmology Society of the UK in 1933.

CAUSATION

This syndrome is inherited as an autosomal dominant. The penetrance rate appears to be high, but the degree to which sufferers are affected is variable. There is a high rate of mutations accounting for this syndrome: about half of all the cases described are thought to be due to this cause. Some of the babies born with Treacher Collins syndrome caused by a new mutation have fathers who are older than normal.

This syndrome has been successfully diagnosed prenatally using fetoscopic methods. The specific characteristics have also been seen on ultrasound screening.

CHARACTERISTICS

The abnormalities seen in Treacher Collins syndrome solely affect the face and associated anatomical structures.

The bones of the **cheeks** (maxillae) are small and underdeveloped. This characteristic gives the false impression that the individual has a large nose, and it is often initially the most noticeable feature.

The **lower jaw** can also be small, giving the appearance of a receding chin. This feature can lead to problems with respiration and feeding during the early days of life. When muscles relax during sleep, the tiny, underdeveloped jaw can drop back, allowing the baby's tongue to fall back into his/her throat, which effectively obstructs breathing. This dangerous problem is most likely to occur if the baby is put to sleep on his/her back. The safest position for these babies is on their sides (laying babies to sleep on their stomachs is thought to be a possible factor in the causation of sudden infant death syndrome, and it should therefore be avoided, even though it would otherwise appear to be an ideal position for the baby with Treacher Collins syndrome).

Feeding can be difficult because of the small jaw. A good "seal" around the nipple is almost impossible to obtain until the baby matures and his/her lower jaw develops further.

Eyes have a downward slant at the outside edge, compounding the unusual appearance of the face. The lower **eyelids** may have a small gap, or "nick," in their length (colomba), and **eyelashes** may be absent on the nasal side of the eye. Fortunately, the colomba never seems to affect any other structures of the eye, as is the case in some other syndromes, such as CHARGE association. There is no visual defect associated with Treacher Collins syndrome.

Ears can be small and malformed. The internal parts of the ears, including the external auditory canal and the middle ear can also be abnormally developed. In around half the children with Treacher Collins syndrome, a conductive deafness occurs as a result of these abnormalities.

Occasionally (in about 28% of cases), the baby with Treacher Collins syndrome may be born with a **cleft palate.** If present, this defect will add to the early feeding difficulties.

A **heart defect** has also occasionally been found with this syndrome.

Due to the abnormalities possible in both upper and lower jaws, there may be problems with proper eruption of **teeth** at a later date.

MANAGEMENT IMPLICATIONS

Early **breathing and feeding difficulties,** if specific abnormalities are severe, will need skilled specialized attention. Nasogastric feeding may be necessary if sucking is impossible in the first few weeks of life. A temporary tracheotomy may be necessary for the most severely affected children.

Surgery may be needed to repair a **cleft palate,** if one is present. Surgery may also be necessary to repair some of the unusual facial features. Great improvement, particularly to the problems in the upper jaw, is possible through plastic surgery.

The most important aspect of care for the child with Treacher Collins syndrome is the early diagnosis of any **conductive deafness** that may arise due to the abnormalities in the auditory system. In the past, children with severe hearing problems were often thought to be mentally retarded, and as a result, both educational facilities and general handling were inappropriate. Hearing aids may be necessary from an early age; this help with hearing will ensure that development is not delayed in other fields.

Orthodontic help may be required later on in childhood if teeth erupt crookedly.

Emotional support from professionals concerned with the welfare of the family may be necessary for both child and parents, especially if the child is teased at school about his/her unusual facial features.

THE FUTURE

Life expectancy is normal. A normal range of career choices is open to the child with Treacher Collins syndrome, unless deafness is a limitation.

Genetic counseling is advisable before pregnancy.

SELF-HELP GROUP

Treacher Collins Foundation
P.O. Box 683
Norwich, VT 05055-0683
802-649-3050 or 800-TCF-2055
http://mcrcr2.med.nyu.edu/murphp01/tcollins.htm

Tuberous Sclerosis

INCIDENCE

The estimated incidence of tuberous sclerosis is between 1 in every 30,000 and 1 in every 40,000 live births. It is thought to account for 0.5% of all children with a significant mental handicap. Boys and girls are affected equally.

HISTORY

Tuberous sclerosis was first recognized in 1880 by Dr. Bournville, who described the pathological changes in the brain. In 1908, Dr. Vogt put together the triad of features, mental retardation, seizures, and the specific type of rash. In 1969, the genetic causation of the condition was described.

Much interest and work, particularly in the USA, has taken place over the past two decades. Research has resulted in greater understanding of the possible long-term effects of the condition.

The name, tuberous sclerosis, is derived from the tuber-like swellings that occur and harden (sclerosis) in various tissues and organs of the body.

CAUSATION

Tuberous sclerosis can be dominantly inherited, but many cases are the result of new mutations. The degree of severity varies widely. In 1987, evidence that the gene for tuberous sclerosis is situated on chromosome 9 was reported.

There is no known prenatal diagnosis. If one of the parents is known to have the condition, ultrasound can be used to detect tumors in the baby's heart as early as the 20th week of pregnancy.

CHARACTERISTICS

Infantile spasms may be the first sign to alert a doctor to a diagnosis of tuberous sclerosis. The spasms are a very specific type of seizure that occurs in early infancy, in which the baby bends at the hips a number of times in very rapid succession. (These attacks are also known as "salaam" attacks.) A characteristic pattern is seen on EEG. Affected children can suffer from seizures throughout life. These seizures can disturb sleep—

creating difficulties when settling down to sleep as well as problems with waking throughout the night.

Skin lesions of a specific nature may be the first sign if seizures do not occur in infancy.

Areas of **lesser pigmentation** than the surrounding skin may occur, often in the shape of an ash leaf. **"Shagreen patches"** (areas of raised, thickened, slightly pigmented skin) also appear, particularly over the lower back.

Later in childhood, the typical **"adenoma sebaceum"** appear round the nose and in a butterfly shape across the cheeks. They can extend to the forehead and chin, but they rarely extend below the neck. In spite of the name, these lesions have nothing to do with the sebaceous glands; they are nevi surrounding the hair follicles.

"Cafe-au-lait" spots, similar to those seen in neurofibromatosis, can also occur, although not in such large numbers as with the latter disease. (Tuberous sclerosis is not connected with neurofibromatosis in any way apart from this common aspect.)

Tumors of varying sizes and types are found in various organs of the body, such as the heart, brain, liver, spleen, bones, and kidneys. Any particular individual with tuberous sclerosis will not be affected with tumors in all of these organs, but the possibility that such growths have occurred must be evaluated when symptoms relating to various bodily systems arise.

Teeth: pitting is often seen in the enamel of the teeth, and fibrous growths can also occur in the gums.

Mental retardation is found in just over half of the children with tuberous sclerosis. The mental handicap is usually obvious by the time the child is two years old. The remaining percentage of children have normal intelligence.

Children with mental handicap due to tuberous sclerosis can exhibit **behavioral problems,** including outbursts of rage and other inappropriate expressions of emotion. When the child reaches adolescence, such problems can be even more difficult to control due to his/her size and physical abilities.

Varying degrees of tuberous sclerosis can occur—for example, only the skin lesions may be visible in a parent of a child with tuberous sclerosis. Silent tumors could be present in the brain or other parts of the body under these circumstances. Recognizing these signs will assist in genetic counseling.

MANAGEMENT IMPLICATIONS

Treatment is symptomatic, as there is no cure for tuberous sclerosis.

Seizures: it is important to control early seizures as far as possible, as such control may possibly prevent the onset of mental handicap. A CAT scan will determine the site of the lesions in the brain (the "tubers" described by Bournville). Similarly, parents of children with tuberous sclerosis who only have the typical skin lesions should also be investigated by CAT scan.

Ultrasound investigation of heart and kidneys is a sensible precaution to exclude lesions in these organs, particularly if there are any related symptoms of cardiac or renal problems.

Follow-up of children with tuberous sclerosis is important, as it will help to diagnose and treat as far as possible any problems relating to potential tumors in various parts of the body.

Mental handicap: it is crucial that the individual child's abilities are assessed, and their development should be reviewed on a regular basis. Schooling must be appropriate to the individual child's needs. Advice to both parents and teachers at each stage is of vital importance. Behavioral problems, if severe, can benefit from the help of a clinical psychologist.

Dental care is important, as the state of the enamel is typically poor.

Genetic counseling of parents who wish to have additional children must be undertaken; the child with tuberous sclerosis should receive similar assistance when he/she reaches reproductive age.

THE FUTURE

Half of the children with tuberous sclerosis will lead normal lives and will only need to be aware of the possibility of manifestations of their condition in a wide variety of organs throughout their body. Children with tuberous sclerosis who have a varying degree of mental handicap will need advice on work prospects, and a few with severe mental handicap will need full-time care throughout their lives.

Life span is dependent upon the presence, or absence, of tumors in various vital organs of the body.

SELF-HELP GROUP

National Tuberous Sclerosis Association
8181 Professional Place, Suite 110
Landover, MD 20785-2226
800-225-6872 or 301-459-9888
http://www.ntsa.org/guests/main.web
email: ntsa@ntsa.org

Turner Syndrome

ALTERNATIVE NAMES

Chromosome 45/X syndrome; Ullrich–Turner syndrome.

INCIDENCE

For approximately every 2,500 live female births, 1 girl will be affected by Turner syndrome. (Only girls are affected, due to the mode of inheritance.) As with all syndromes, there are a wide range of features that, when put together, add up to a specific syndrome. Sufferers from Turner syndrome will not necessarily show all these features, but there will be sufficient evidence to support a clinical diagnosis of Turner syndrome.

HISTORY

Turner syndrome was first defined by Dr. Henry Turner in 1938. This American doctor described four of the clinical features—small stature, lack of sexual development, a webbed neck, and a wide-carrying angle at the elbows—in adult women. It was later found that these women had high levels of gonadotropins in their urine, together with a complete lack of ovarian tissue. Those vital sexual organs are replaced by whorls of connective tissue.

It was not until 1959 that the genetic background to the condition was demonstrated.

CAUSATION

Girls with Turner syndrome have only 45 chromosomes instead of the usual full complement of 46. The chromosome missing is one of the X chromosomes. (XX denotes a female and XY a male. Girls with Turner syndrome are denoted as XO). However, some girls with Turner syndrome have a "mosaic" chromosomal pattern, that is, some cells have the full complement of sex chromosomes. Such chromosome patterns are denoted as XO/XX. The pattern can be reflected in the clinical picture.

As 99% of girls with Turner syndrome are infertile, there is small chance of the condition being inherited from the female side. The missing chromosome is lost during cell division. In the literature, there are 54 reported pregnancies in women with Turner syndrome. The outcome of these pregnancies has been variable; more than half of the babies were miscarried or stillborn. A few pregnancies have resulted in the birth of normal children.

Prenatal diagnosis is available by chorionic villus sampling and/or amniocentesis

CHARACTERISTICS

Short stature is the most consistent and obvious problem. Growth is usually within normal limits until around three years of age, although the baby may be significantly shorter than normal at birth. After growth slows, the girl with Turner syndrome will progressively fall behind her peers in height. This failure to grow is also very marked during the early teenage years, when the normal growth spurt of puberty occurs. Special charts to plot the growth of girls with Turner syndrome are available. Final height will be a maximum of 5 feet (150 centimeters), but more usually, height does not surpass 4 feet 8 inches (141 centimeters). Treatment may assist the girl in gaining a few inches.

Fertility: Due to the nondevelopment of the ovaries, all girls with true Turner syndrome will be unable to conceive. Also as a result of this ovarian problem, puberty can be a difficult time, as secondary sexual characteristics fail to develop without treatment. Breasts do not develop; pubic hair does not appear; and menstruation does not occur.

Heart: girls with Turner syndrome are more likely than their peers to suffer from coarctation (narrowing) of the aorta. As a result of this condition, affected girls may have raised blood pressure and peripheral vascular problems later in life unless treatment is given. Other heart anomalies can also occur.

Eyes: There is a higher incidence than normal of visual problems (either near- or far-sightedness), for which glasses may be necessary. Lazy eye is also more common, and epicanthic folds and drooping eyelids (ptosis) can give a false impression of sleepiness.

Ears: Girls with Turner syndrome often suffer frequently from otitis media, which can lead to a conductive deafness if not adequately treated.

Intelligence is usually normal in girls with Turner syndrome, but some may have specific learning difficulties. For example, number concepts can pose problems, although reading, vocabulary, and visual memory skills are good.

Thyroid function: There is a higher incidence than normal of hypothyroidism, due to lymphocytic thyroiditis, in Turner syndrome.

The following added features may, or may not, be seen.

- **Webbing of the neck** is a fairly common feature, and it may be one of the first diagnostic clues in infancy. Loose folds of skin may also be seen in the nape of the neck in the young baby.
- **Swelling of the backs of the hands and feet** is also common during infancy, due to faulty lymphatic drainage. This condition may persist throughout life.
- A **broad chest** with widely spaced nipples is a fairly consistent feature.
- There is a wide-carrying angle at the **elbows.**
- **Low-set ears** can be a feature.
- A **high-arched palate** can occur, with the result that the teeth may be overcrowded.
- A **shortened fourth finger** is seen in 50% of girls with Turner syndrome.

All these latter features are coincidental findings, which may, or may not, be present in girls with Turner syndrome. Few of them cause problems, but, if present, they can assist clinical diagnosis.

MANAGEMENT IMPLICATIONS

Given the complete lack of ovarian tissue, nothing can be done medically to alter the **infertile state.** Much can be done, however, to ensure that **secondary sexual characteristics** develop normally. At puberty, around 12 to 13 years, estrogen in some form is given. This hormone will ensure breast development, the growth of pubic hair, and the maturation of the uterus to a normal size. The vaginal epithelium also matures. When these changes are fully under way, cyclical treatment with the appropriate hormone is started. This treatment will ensure that menstruation occurs regularly, although, of course, without ovulation. Treatment must continue at least until the natural menopausal age.

Short stature: growth hormone and/or steroids can be given; such drugs can help in many cases to increase final height, but in spite of this treatment, final height is never more than 5 feet. Lack of height may present educational problems as schooling progresses. Physical education, in particular, can often be difficult for shorter children. Care must be taken not to treat girls with Turner syndrome as younger than they really are just because of their lack of inches or their lack of secondary sexual characteristics.

Coarctation of the aorta, if present, must be corrected surgically. This abnormality should be discovered at routine developmental checks when femoral pulses are found to be diminished.

Eyes: continuing checks must be made for refractory errors, and glasses prescribed where necessary. Lazy eye should be corrected, both to prevent amblyopia and for cosmetic purposes.

Ears: Frequent bouts of otitis media should be adequately treated and hearing tested regularly after each severe infection. Chronic otitis media is common and may require myringotomy and the insertion of ventilation tubes. School teachers should be made aware of potential problems in this area.

Feeding problems can occur in infancy in Turner syndrome. The cause for such difficulties is not clear, but symptomatic treatment and support will ensure that babies grow satisfactorily through this phase.

Watch must be maintained throughout life for signs of **hypothyroidism**—unusual weight gain, slowness of action and speech, hoarse voice, dry skin, and scanty hair. Replacement therapy with thyroxine may be indicated under these conditions.

Specific **learning difficulties** may occur, particularly in word comprehension and presentation. There may also be difficulties with mathematical concepts. Intelligence is generally normal, but there may be mild retardation. There may also be spatial difficulties with large movements, such as throwing and catching balls. Fine movements, such as those used in painting, drawing, and sewing, are all usually within normal limits. These latter tasks should therefore be encouraged, and help should be offered to avoid upset and frustration with other activities that are not as easily pursued.

THE FUTURE

Girls with Turner syndrome can expect a normal life span. The inability to have children through ordinary methods of fertilization can cause great sadness, but in vitro fertilization by donor ova is possible as the uterus is normal. Adoption and foster parenting are also possibilities.

Sexual feelings and relationships are normal, as the vagina and uterus are of normal size.

Clothes may be a problem when small-sized apparel is only available in styles that are less mature than those worn by the girl's peers. Also, girls with Turner syndrome tend to put on weight easily as they get older, making it even more difficult to find appropriate clothing. Dressmaking at home is a good option to pursue.

SELF-HELP GROUP

Turner's Syndrome Society of the United States
1313 Southeast 5th Street, Suite 327
Minneapolis, MN 55414
800-365-9944
http://www.turner-syndrome-us.org

Usher Syndrome

INCIDENCE

Reports on the incidence of this syndrome vary greatly. In 1987, the number of people suffering from Usher syndrome was thought to be only about 5 in every 100,000, but a much higher incidence has been estimated in populations in Finland, Norway, and parts of the USA.

Boys and girls can be equally affected. Among children in schools for the profoundly deaf, Usher syndrome is to be found in as many as 10% of these children, which indicates that it is an important cause of severe hearing loss.

Some children who have been diagnosed as having Usher syndrome also show signs of mental instability and/or mental retardation. When these added problems are noted, the disorder is termed Hallgren syndrome. The exact connection between these two syndromes is not clear.

CAUSATION

Usher syndrome is inherited in an autosomally recessive manner. Some children have the added disability of poor balance. This condition may be a variant of Usher syndrome, or it may have a different basic cause with possible different modes of inheritance.

Abnormalities in the levels of polyunsaturated fatty acids have recently been found; this evidence suggests that Usher syndrome may yet prove to be a metabolic disorder.

There is no prenatal test available, but gene mapping is proceeding.

CHARACTERISTICS

Usher syndrome mainly affects two systems of the body—hearing and vision. (The exception to this statement, of course, occurs when the other problems associated with Hallgren syndrome are present.)

Hearing: 90% of babies with Usher syndrome are born with a profound hearing loss. It is important that this severe problem is detected as soon as possible so that appropriate action can be taken early. Hearing tests on newborn babies are ideal. Later routine tests of hearing—at around seven to nine months of age—will also pick up deafness, but parents may suspect that their babies are not hearing properly long before that age, and testing should take place earlier if that is the case. When babies show a lack of response to loud sudden noises or delays in response to voices, all care givers should consider the possibility of a congenital deafness. The deafness in Usher syndrome is of a sensorineural type.

If Usher syndrome has been diagnosed in a close family member, any suspicion of deafness in a new member must be taken seriously.

Vision is normal at birth in the baby with Usher syndrome and remains so for the first few years of life. At around ten years of age, the child may discover that he/she is unable to see as well in the dark as his/her contemporaries. Peripheral vision may also begin to become limited. Loss of peripheral vision, which can be suspected if the child is becoming unaware of objects or people beside him/her when looking straight ahead, is due to pigmentation of the retina. In Usher syndrome, in particular, "spicule" concretions of abnormal pigment are laid down in the retina. Other pathological changes are also seen in this part of the eye, and along with the abnormal retinal pigmentation, these factors are responsible for a much reduced visual acuity. Vision will become gradually more and more reduced until complete blindness is the result. This tragedy occurs certainly before the middle years of life, and in many cases at an earlier age.

Glaucoma, a dangerously high pressure inside the eyeball, can also occur in Usher syndrome, and must be remembered when caring for a child with this condition. The signs of glaucoma are pain in the eye, rapid blurring of vision, and in some cases, the seeing of "haloes" around sources of light.

Cataracts can also add to the visual problems of sufferers from Usher syndrome.

About 10% of children with Usher syndrome will have minimal hearing and visual problems in early childhood. By puberty, however, their hearing loss becomes obvious and gradually worsens, and the pigmentation of the retina makes its appearance, so that vision also regrettably declines.

Given the relatively high frequency of Usher syndrome among profoundly deaf children, night and peripheral vision should be checked in all severely deaf children.

Ataxia, or poor balance, is sometimes also associated with Usher syndrome. Children with this manifestation will, for example, find it difficult to turn quickly or balance on one foot—movements that their peers can easily perform. This problem does not always occur, but it can be an added factor to be remembered when the diagnosis of Usher syndrome is suspected.

MANAGEMENT IMPLICATIONS

Deafness, if present from birth, will require a full audiometric assessment to quantify the exact amount of hearing loss. Early teaching is vital for the development of any speech, and specialist teachers of the deaf must be involved early.

Vision also requires full assessment early in the child's life to establish a base line for his/her visual acuity at that time. Regular routine checks, particularly on night and peripheral vision, should be done on all profoundly deaf children. Night vision lenses can be helpful in the initial stages of the abnormal pigmentation of the retina. Other aids for failing vision will become necessary later, and blindness will eventually need specialized help.

Cataracts, if present, should be removed to maximize any residual vision.

Glaucoma must also be remembered as a possibility and treated if found to be present.

Parents will need sensitive and continuing counseling concerning the likely outcome of their child's inherited condition. Feelings of guilt must be allayed, and help given to minimize the effects of disturbed vision and hearing as they arise.

Schooling should be geared toward vocational training helpful for deaf and/or blind adults. This approach may seem very hard to take at a time when the child still has some residual vision left, but given the progressive nature of the disorder, it is important that all steps should be taken to reduce the impact of blindness when it does occur.

THE FUTURE

The future can be difficult for persons with Usher syndrome. Most people will be severely handicapped, both visually and auditorally, by the time early adulthood is reached. Specialized training and teaching in the early days can reduce later problems. Full explanation of the probable outcome should be given to parents, and to the individuals with Usher syndrome when it is felt that they are ready to receive this information.

Usher syndrome does not reduce life span. Genetic counseling will be necessary when reproductive age is reached.

SELF-HELP GROUP

Usher Family Support
4918 42nd Avenue, S
Minneapolis, MN 55417
612-724-6982
email: kadbmn@aol.com

VATER Association

INCIDENCE

An "association" is a grouping of abnormalities arising together more often than is probable by chance. Many systems or organs of the body can be affected by VATER association; the name is an acronym of the parts of the body affected.

VATER association is diagnosed when three of the six possible abnormalities are present: *v*ertebral abnormality; *a*nal malformation; *tra*chea defects; *e*sophageal defects; *r*enal problems; and *r*adial limb defects.

There are several hundred known persons suffering from this specific association of abnormalities, which was first described in 1973. It is thought that VATER association is not always recognized as such. Many babies previously described as having "multiple abnormalities" could well have had the specific grouping of VATER association.

Boys and girls are affected in equal numbers.

This condition is more often seen in the children of diabetic mothers.

CAUSATION

The wide-ranging, and often severe, abnormalities of this association of defects could point to a chromosomal abnormality, but no unusual chromosome pattern has been identified in VATER association.

Most cases have arisen out of the blue, but a few families with more than one affected member are known. Genetic counseling and family studies are advisable after the birth of a baby with this particular grouping of defects.

There is no prenatal test for this condition, although if there are bony abnormalities in the arms, these can be visualized during scanning in the pregnancy.

CHARACTERISTICS

Vertebral abnormalities can take many forms, ranging from the vertebrae being fused together to only half a vertebra being present. These defects are more often found in the lower part of the body, in the lumbar region. Extra vertebrae are occasionally present: for example, there may be six or seven lumbar vertebrae instead of the usual five. This excess of vertebrae can also occur higher up the spine, in the thoracic region. Here also, extra ribs can be sometimes seen in association with the extra vertebrae. The effects of these abnormalities depend very much on the site and severity of the defect. Sometimes, these unusual features are only noted when an X-ray examination is done for another, quite separate, reason.

Anal atresia: in the severest form of the association, there is only a dimpling of the skin where the anus should be situated. The lower bowel can be normally formed, but it does not extend as far as the exterior. Sometimes the anal canal and anus are present, but they are very much narrowed and function only with difficulty.

Tracheal defect: the extent and severity of this abnormality can vary. The most severe problems arise when there is an opening (a fistula) between the esophagus and the trachea. In conjunction with the fistula, the esophagus itself can be small and under developed. The baby with this type of defect will have severe respiratory problems at birth. Swallowing will also present major difficulties; the extent of this problem varies with the severity of the anatomical defect.

Renal abnormalities can also occur, and they vary in severity and type. Kidneys may be situated in unusual positions in the abdomen, and "horseshoe" kidneys are relatively common. Again, effects will vary according to the actual abnormality. In the most severe cases, renal failure is a distinct possibility in the infant's early days.

Radial limb abnormalities: the radius is one of the bones of the forearm, and in some babies with VATER association, this bone is of a small size or it can be absent altogether. This defect can be detected by prenatal scanning.

Heart defects are also occasionally present in this particular association.

For a definite diagnosis of VATER association to be made, three of the described abnormalities must be present. It must be emphasized that the degree of the abnormalities, and hence the severity of their effects, can vary enormously.

MANAGEMENT IMPLICATIONS

Respiratory difficulties will be the most apparent problem immediately after birth, and they may create an urgent need for special care facilities. Depending on the degree of abnormality, emergency surgery to correct the anatomical defects may be necessary.

Feeding problems may also occur at a slightly later date if the defect in the trachea is connected to the esophagus.

Renal abnormalities can present serious problems in the neonatal period if the defects are severe. Renal failure is a distinct possibility in some of the babies who have a severe renal abnormality. These babies will need special care facilities.

A **narrowed or absent anus** will require surgical correction in the early days of life.

If the baby can survive all these potential major surgical procedures, and the defects are not so severe as to be irreparable, the outlook is surprisingly good, although renal failure is a continuing possible threat if the kidney abnormalities are present and severe.

The **vertebral** and other possible **bony abnormalities** may give rise to a few problems of mobility later in life. Again, surgical intervention may be needed for proper function. The absence or defective size of the radius in the arm can cause problems of rotation movements, as well as difficulties in carrying anything weighty on this arm.

THE FUTURE

It is difficult to be specific about the future for a baby born with VATER association. The range of severity and types of defect is so wide that some individuals will be able to lead nearly normal lives, while others may be severely physically handicapped.

It is rare for the central nervous system to be affected in any way, and intellectual function is only very rarely affected. In this regard, career choices will be wide.

Life span is also dependent on the type and severity of the abnormalities found.

SELF-HELP GROUPS

TEF/VATER Support Network
15301 Grey Fox Road
Upper Marlboro, MD 20772
301-952-6837

VATER Association
520 Greensboro Street
Startville, MD 39759
601-323-1951

The VATER Connection
1722 Yucca Lane
Emporia, KS 66801
316-342-6954
http://www.vaterconnection.org
email: angie@vaterconnection.org

Vitiligo

ALTERNATIVE NAMES

Primary achromia; idiopathic leukoderma.

INCIDENCE

This skin condition can occur at any time of life, but around 50% of cases occur in children before the teenage years. Two separate studies have suggested that the incidence can be as high as 1 in every 200 people; the amount of skin surface affected varies greatly from person to person.

Both sexes are thought to be equally affected.

CAUSATION

The exact cause for this skin condition is not known. Some authorities consider it to be an auto-immune disease. If a number of family members are affected, the risk to a child born to a mother who herself has vitiligo is thought to be 50%.

The basic pathology of vitiligo is an absence of melanocytes (the cells in the skin associated with pigmentation) in the areas of skin affected. The reason for this loss is unknown.

CHARACTERISTICS

A varying amount of **skin**—anywhere on the body—can be affected by vitiligo. These areas of skin are completely white. In the most severe cases, half of the body surface has the typical loss of pigment. In children with a dark complexion, this feature stands out in sharp contrast to the normally colored skin.

No other characteristics are known to be associated with this skin condition. It is important, however, to exclude any other auto-immune conditions—such as those affecting the thyroid gland, adrenal glands, or stomach—as auto-immune conditions frequently affect more than one part of the body.

MANAGEMENT IMPLICATIONS

It is important to protect the depigmented areas of skin against **sunburn.** With no protective melanin in the skin, severe burning can result from even limited exposure to sunlight.

Sunscreen creams with a high protection factor (SPF) need to be used for even brief exposure to the sun. It must also be remembered that sunburn can occur even on a cloudy, but bright, day.

Children can be unkind to classmates with vitiligo. Some sensitive children will respond to this form of **teasing** with a variety of behavioral patterns ranging from school phobia to aggressive behavior.

It is important that teachers are aware of the **noninfectious** nature of vitiligo. (Vitiligo can be confused at times with pityriasis alba—a skin condition, probably viral, in which areas of skin temporarily lose pigmentation. This condition will clear up within a few weeks with no treatment, whereas vitiligo is a long-lasting condition.)

For small areas of depigmented skin, **cosmetic creams** can be used, but this approach is impracticable for larger areas of affected skin.

THE FUTURE

Most cases of vitiligo are life-long, although spontaneous remission can very occasionally occur.

It is important to remember that the depigmented areas of skin are more prone to skin cancers, especially in climates that have long days of hot sunshine.

SELF-HELP GROUP

National Vitiligo Foundation
611 South Fleishel Avenue
Tyler, TX 75701
903-531-0074
http://www.nvfi.org/menu.htm
email: vitiligo@trimofran.org

Waardenburg Syndrome

This syndrome has three distinct subtypes, depending on the presence, and severity, of the specific characteristics. For example, type 3 has abnormalities of the limbs in addition to the features shown by the other two types. The general overall incidence of the condition, taking all the subtypes into account, is between 1 birth in every 20,000 and 1 birth in every 40,000.

The importance of this syndrome lies in the fact that among children who are deaf from birth, 3 in every 100 have Waardenburg syndrome.

CAUSATION

Waardenburg syndrome is inherited as an autosomal dominant condition. In a few families having a specific variant of the condition, the inheritance pattern is thought to be a recessive one. There is also some link with a particular form of albinism in that variant.

Both boys and girls can be equally affected. It is probable that the affected gene is located on chromosome 9. There is no prenatal test available for Waardenburg syndrome.

CHARACTERISTICS

All the characteristics of Waardenburg syndrome—apart from the limb abnormalities of type 3—are confined to the head and neck region.

Almost all children with Waardenburg syndrome have a specific unusual finding in the shape of their eyes. The inner edge of the eye, instead of being tight up against the bridge of the nose, is displaced outward. This positioning affects the openings of the lower tear ducts, which are also placed farther away from the midline of the face than is usual. While this positioning leads to few problems, tears tend to flow less easily than normal.

Eyes can have other very specific striking characteristics. In a percentage of children with Waardenburg syndrome, one eye can be light blue in color, while the other eye can be dark brown, if that is the characteristic eye color of the child's family. The two different eye colors can give a most unusual aspect to the appearance of the face. In some instances, only a small segment of the iris is of a lighter color, but that is still a noticeable characteristic. This feature has no effect on vision.

The only possible visual difficulty seen in Waardenburg syndrome can be the onset of **glaucoma,** a dangerous increase in tension inside the eyeball. This condition probably occurs when the unusual structure of the orbit makes normal drainage of fluid from the eye difficult.

The **noses** of children with Waardenburg syndrome are small at birth and tend to remain so throughout life. This feature can lead to young children in particular having a frequently blocked nose, with more frequent upper respiratory tract infections than usual being the norm. These children are often "mouth breathers."

Along with the unusual eye shape and tiny noses goes an unusual eyebrow feature. **Eyebrows** tend to grow across the forehead until they meet in the middle over the bridge of the nose. Of course, not everyone with confluent eyebrows has Waardenburg syndrome, but this feature is yet one more sign that can confirm a diagnosis of the syndrome.

Hair: one of the most striking features of Waardenburg syndrome (especially when occurring in conjunction with different colored eyes) is a completely white "forelock." This trait can be present at birth, even in a baby with a dark head of hair. Occasionally, this unusual coloring disappears during early childhood, only to reappear again during the teenage years. Early graying of all facial hair, eyebrows, and eyelashes as well as the hair on the head, has also been reported; graying can occur not just in the twenties but as early as seven years of age!

Deafness is the most serious of the features of Waardenburg syndrome. This characteristic affects up to one-quarter of all sufferers from the condition. The deafness is present from birth, and it can affect both ears or only one. It is a sensorineural type, in which the actual nerves of hearing are affected. It is vitally important that the deafness is recognized early so that speech, as well as many other aspects of normal development, are not secondarily affected. In the past, some profoundly deaf children were labeled mentally retarded—and treated as such. With today's knowledge of normal child development and screening procedures, this regrettable mistake should never occur.

These are the usual signs of all the types of Waardenburg syndrome. Children with type 3 may have, in addition, developmental abnormalities of their **upper limbs,** which may take the form of a generalized lack of prenatal growth of arms. Alternatively, there may be abnormalities of the fingers; extra fingers may be present, or two or more fingers can be fused together. With such deformities, of course, there will be problems of fine, precise movement.

MANAGEMENT IMPLICATIONS

It is important to recognize Waardenburg syndrome early in a child's life so hearing and vision can be checked.

Routine checks on **hearing** from an early age should identify any hearing loss. Serious note should always be taken when parents suggest that their baby is not hearing properly. Very special care must be taken, under these circumstances, to check hearing thoroughly at regular intervals. If the baby is profoundly deaf, referral to a service for hearing impaired children (if available) is important. Early help is vital if speech is to be attained at all. Later in childhood, special educational facilities for deaf children may be needed if the deafness is bilateral and profound. Children with lesser degrees of hearing loss may also need speech therapy, as well as complete hearing assessment.

Vision: glaucoma may pose a danger to the child's sight. Pain in the child's eyes, blurred vision, or reports of "haloes" around lights indicate the need for urgent visual assessment. Eye drops or surgery will be necessary if the pressure in the eye is found to be raised.

THE FUTURE

The future will largely depend on the presence, or lack, of hearing problems. If deafness is not present, the other features of eye color, white forelock, and unusual eye-shape will point to a lesser manifestation of the syndrome. All these latter characteristics will have no bearing on either career choice or leisure activities—in fact, they can be added attractive features! In some instances, the more minor aspects of Waardenburg syndrome are only recognized after a more severely affected family member has been investigated.

SELF-HELP GROUPS

There are no known organizations dedicated specifically to Waardenburg syndrome, but the following groups may be able to offer assistance.

National Organization for Rare Disorders (NORD)
P.O. Box 8923
New Fairfield, CT 06812-8923
203-746-6518 or 800-999-6673
http://www.nord-rdb.com/~orphan
email: orphan@nord-rdb.com

National Association of the Deaf
814 Thayer Avenue, Suite 250
Silver Spring, MD 20910-4500
301-587-1788
http://www.nad.org
email: NADinfo@nad.org

American Foundation for the Blind
11 Penn Plaza, Suite 300
New York, NY 10001
212-502-7600
http://www.afb.org
email: afbinfo@afb.org

West Syndrome

ALTERNATIVE NAMES

Infantile spasms; hypsarrhythmia.

INCIDENCE

The exact incidence of West syndrome is difficult to determine, as it merges with the many other types of epilepsy. It is only when specific tests are carried out, and the results added to the typical clinical signs, that this syndrome can be identified.

CAUSATION

This syndrome is caused by the baby's immature brain reacting to any one of a number of factors, including a lack of oxygen at birth, infections (such as meningitis) in the early days of life, or some injury to the brain. In a significant number of babies with West syndrome, some developmental abnormality in the brain is also found.

Other possible causes of this particular syndrome include some disturbances of metabolism, which in turn have an effect on the young brain. Examples of this type of cause are phenylketonuria (in which there is abnormal metabolism of the amino acid); phenylalanine; hypoglycemia (in which blood sugar levels are low for some reason); or low levels of pyridoxine (a vitamin of the B group).

Each of these factors can cause a failure of development of the normal organization of the electrical activity of the brain. This problem results in the typical seizures seen in West syndrome.

Obviously, in many cases of West syndrome, there is no direct inheritance pattern involved (for example, if the cause is an infection or the lack of oxygen at a critical time). When the cause is found to be metabolic, the most usual pattern of inheritance is autosomal recessive.

CHARACTERISTICS

Babies with West syndrome usually have no problems at birth. However, if the birth has been difficult, and oxygen lack is a marked feature, these problems may be one of the precipitating causes for the condition.

Some authorities describe two distinct types of the syndrome: one that occurs before six months of age (about 10% of the cases), and one that occurs after that age. The latter type is thought to be due possibly to an unrecognized case of encephalitis or to an underlying defect in the metabolism in the brain. In the latter type, the child subsequently has good motor skills, but she/he often has difficulties with language.

Seizures of a specific nature will begin to occur at any time between the early neonatal days and two years old. The most usual time of onset is between three and eight months old. The baby will jerk into a flexed position and then rapidly return to the normal way of lying. These seizures can occur in rapid succession. Sometimes, it is only the baby's head that is involved, a nodding motion being the only indication that a seizure is occurring. This type of seizure is also known as hypsarrythmia, and it can be identified on an EEG tracing. Sixty percent of babies with West syndrome show this typical tracing when an EEG is recorded.

Before the onset of the seizures, the baby may be developing normally, showing all the usual developmental steps of smiling, head control, etc., in a normal sequence. Other babies with the syndrome may exhibit some developmental delay before seizures first occur.

One fairly frequent feature that is noticed to precede a seizure is a decrease in the baby's **visual alertness.** He/she will not respond as readily to visual stimuli as do babies of a similar age or, indeed, as quickly as he/she had done previously.

The spasms, or seizures, commonly occur shortly after the baby awakes from sleep, and a rapid succession of seizures may follow the first one. CAT scans have shown that 60% of babies with West syndrome have some abnormality of the brain, which can range from a generalized atrophy of this organ to specific abnormalities in certain parts of the brain (cf. Aicardi syndrome).

It is important to exclude a metabolic cause for this syndrome. Specific tests for metabolic disease should be done (for example, tests for abnormalities in the metabolism of certain amino acids and for pyridoxine).

Treatment to control the frequent spasms is with ACTH. This treatment can effectively control the seizures, but relapse can occur, giving rise to the need for a further course of ACTH.

The outlook for babies with West syndrome varies. Ten percent of babies initially suffering this type of seizure will develop normally and have no permanent after-effects. The remainder will be left with varying degrees of mental handicap, and 50% of these children will develop other types of seizures as they get older.

There are no other developmental abnormalities to be seen with West syndrome.

MANAGEMENT IMPLICATIONS

It is important that West syndrome is diagnosed as early as possible, so that a course of treatment can begin. The seizures are quite specific clinically, and the EEG tracing will confirm the type of seizure is that found in West syndrome.

Developmental checks should be routinely performed, preferably by a multidisciplinary team, throughout the early childhood years. Specific areas of delay can then be helped by physical therapy and speech therapy and by other forms of treatment. Specialized teaching in the pre-school years is also valuable for instructing the child in self-help skills.

Schooling will need to be geared to the abilities of each individual child.

Children who subsequently develop other types of seizures will need assessment to determine the best **anticonvulsant drug**, or combination of drugs, necessary to control the seizures.

Parents will need sensitive **counseling** and information about the probable cause behind their child's illness. If possible, short-term nursing care for the child should be arranged so parents and any other children in the family can have a vacation together without the continual worry of caring for a handicapped family member.

THE FUTURE

Ten percent of the children who have West syndrome as babies will be able to lead normal lives with no sequelae following their difficult first days of life. Genetic counseling is advisable once reproductive age is reached. The remainder of children with this syndrome will regrettably have varying degrees of mental handicap for the rest of their lives. Such disabilities will, of course, influence any choice of career, and the most severely handicapped will need full-time care for the rest of their lives.

Life expectancy is within the normal range.

SELF-HELP GROUP

Epilepsy Foundation of America
4351 Garden City Drive
Landover, MD 20785
301-459-3700
http://www.efa.org/
email: webmaster@efa.org

Williams Syndrome

ALTERNATIVE NAME

Infantile hypercalcemia.

INCIDENCE

Estimates of number of babies suffering from this syndrome have only recently been reported: incidence is thought to be in the region of 1 in every 10,000 births. Boys and girls can be affected equally.

CAUSATION

Williams syndrome was thought to arise only as a sporadic new mutation, but it has recently been suggested that the condition may be inherited as an autosomal dominant.

The basic pathology is one of a fault in calcium metabolism, which leads to an excess of calcium in the body as a whole. The build-up of calcium, if not corrected, can affect brain cells and lead to a degree of mental handicap.

CHARACTERISTICS

Facial features are quite typical for all individuals with Williams syndrome. Boys and girls with this syndrome will have round, chubby faces with full lips and a tip-tilted nose.

During infancy, babies with Williams syndrome often **fail to grow** at the normal rate. Their birth weight is often on the low side, and they grow slowly, usually along, or below, the third percentile line on the standard growth charts. Excessive vomiting can also be a feature, and that condition adds to the problems of adequate weight gain.

Sleeping, too, can be a problem. Parents can become completely worn out by their restless, demanding baby who, in addition to not gaining weight along the usual lines, does not seem to want to sleep. This sleeplessness continues into later childhood.

Along with the lack of a normal sleep pattern goes a good deal of **hyperactivity** during the day, making it even more difficult for parents to get adequate rest.

Behavioral problems are commonly seen, and as the child with Williams syndrome gets older, he/she becomes increasingly verbally able. Verbal acuity can add to the parents' problems, as, at first sight, the child appears to be older and more able than is really the case. All in all, children with Williams syndrome can be extraordinarily difficult to handle.

Heart defects frequently occur; the most often seen abnormality is aortic stenosis—a narrowing of the large blood vessel leaving the heart. Other structural defects in the cardiovascular system are also seen more often than is usual.

Hearing: it has been reported that children with Williams syndrome seem to be especially susceptible to loud noise and find any excess of noise very distressing.

A further possible complication of the high calcium levels found in this condition is that the child, at a comparatively early age, may suffer from **renal calculi,** or kidney stones, those accretions of calcium that can be excruciatingly painful as they pass down the ureters into the bladder.

MANAGEMENT IMPLICATIONS

The **failure to thrive** in infancy must be patiently treated to ensure that the baby obtains adequate nutrition in spite of the persistent vomiting and general hyperactive behavior. Dietary advice is essential to know which are the most suitable foods to offer the baby with Williams syndrome. For example, foods low in vitamin D and calcium are advisable if high levels of calcium in the blood persist. The early difficulties with feeding usually improve with maturity, although episodes of hypercalcemia can recur in later life. Nevertheless, many children with Williams syndrome do not achieve a normal adult height, always remaining on the short side of normal.

Heart defects, if severe and causing symptoms, may require cardiac surgery. The ongoing care of a cardiologist is always advisable.

Education will very much depend on the child's abilities, and on the extent of his/her behavioral problems. Individual educational programs, best suited to each child's range of ability, are the ideal. Activities that use up some of the abundant energy seen in the child with Williams syndrome are a must. Shorter than normal periods of teaching will accommodate the child's short attention span and also allow time for his/her verbal loquacity. It is all too easy to think of the child with Williams syndrome as more able than he/she really is, due to the extreme ease with which he/she uses words and language. It is only when concepts need to be put into practice that the child will find difficulty.

THE FUTURE

Career choices must be carefully evaluated for people with Williams syndrome. His/her undoubted verbal abilities must not be allowed to hide the true nature of the young person's problems as he/she attempts to cope with the stresses of the adult world.

Life expectancy can be limited by cardiac defects or by the side effects of the high calcium levels in the body, such as the renal problems.

SELF-HELP GROUP

Williams Syndrome Foundation
University of California
Irvine, CA 92679-2310
949-824-7259
http://www.wsf.org

Wolf–Hirshhorn Syndrome

ALTERNATIVE NAMES

Wolf syndrome; partial chromosome 4 deletion syndrome.

INCIDENCE

Wolf–Hirshhorn syndrome is a very rare syndrome, but around 120 cases have been confirmed in the literature. Of these cases, two-thirds have been girls, although babies of either sex can be affected. A number of still-born babies have also found to be affected by this chromosomal defect.

HISTORY

Both Wolf and Hirschhorn described this syndrome in 1965.

CAUSATION

Wolf–Hirschhorn syndrome results from the loss of some of the genetic material on the short arm of chromosome 4. In most cases, this abnormality arises spontaneously, but in around 10% of cases, the syndrome arises as the result of a "balanced translocation." It is important that the parent's chromosomes are examined for the presence of this translocation as future pregnancies may also be affected.

Parental age seems to have no effect on the occurrence of this syndrome.

Chorionic villus sampling can detect this condition in the baby if performed between the 9th and 12th weeks of pregnancy.

CHARACTERISTICS

The baby with Wolf–Hirschhorn syndrome will have a **low birth weight,** even though the pregnancy continued to the full 40 weeks. The lack of adequate growth continues after birth; weight gain occurs very slowly in spite of adequate feeding.

The **facial features** of the baby are quite distinctive, and include:

- a small head—**microcephaly;**

- there is no usual indentation of the **nose** between the eyebrows; instead, there is a continuous line from the forehead to the tip of the nose. This feature has been graphically described as resembling a Greek helmet, the flat bridge of the baby's nose closely resembles the protective nose-piece of this ancient piece of armor;
- **eyes** are widely spaced, and the child may also have a lazy eye;
- the **upper lip** is short;
- the **ears** are low-set.

The baby with Wolf–Hirschhorn syndrome will be **floppy** at birth, and muscle tone will always be weak. Milestones of motor movement will usually be delayed.

Seizures are a frequent occurrence and can be difficult to control.

Learning difficulties are usually severe.

Other characteristics can also be present, although they do not necessarily occur in every baby with this syndrome.

- **Heart defects,** of different types, can occur;
- a **cleft palate and/or lip** can be an immediately obvious feature;
- the **testes** can be small and undescended, and a hypospadias can be present.

MANAGEMENT IMPLICATIONS

Feeding difficulties and **lack of weight gain** can be worrying problems during the early days of life. These problems are due to the baby's poor muscle tone as well as a continuation of the prenatal pattern of inadequate growth. Also, if a cleft palate and/or lip is present, the feeding difficulties are magnified by these anatomical features.

Small, frequent feeds will initially be necessary, and an early referral to a specialist for the best method of treatment of the cleft palate/lip is advisable. Nasogastric feeding may be necessary for some severely affected babies.

Any **heart defect** will need to be diagnosed and assessed, and appropriate treatment should be pursued if heart failure occurs at any time during the early days of life.

Surgical treatment for the **cleft palate** and/or **lip,** if they are present, will need to be organized. The timing of these operative procedures will depend on the physical health of the baby.

Seizures will need to be controlled with anticonvulsant drugs. In many cases, finding the right drug—or combination of drugs—can prove difficult. Several drugs may need to be tried before the most helpful one is found.

Regular **developmental checks** must be carried out to determine the level of mental retardation as well as the development of motor skills. When school age is reached, the appropriate schooling for each individual child needs to be determined with the help of both health and education authorities.

At a later date, the **hypospadias,** if present, will need to be corrected surgically if problems are encountered by the boy being unable to direct the flow of urine.

Genetic counseling is of importance if the parents are considering further pregnancies. If a balanced translocation is found, investigations at an early stage in a future pregnancy will be needed.

THE FUTURE

Many babies with the most profound defects do not survive the first year of life, but if they do, a life of severe handicap will be the regrettable outlook. The average life span is not known, but the teenage years can certainly be attained, and adults with this syndrome have been reported.

An independent life style can unfortunately never be attained.

SELF-HELP GROUP

4p- Support Group
c/o Larry and Sherry Bentley
P.O. Box 1676
Gresham, OR 97030
503-661-1855
email: lbentley@orednet.org *or* lbent503@aol.com

Zollinger–Ellison Syndrome

ALTERNATIVE NAMES

Endocrine neoplasia; Wermer syndrome.

INCIDENCE

The incidence of this rare disorder is not exactly known, but it is comparatively widely reported in the literature. Younger children only infrequently show signs of the condition, but after around ten years of age, signs and symptoms can occur; they can also be delayed into adulthood.

Both boys and girls can be affected

There are a number of conditions that have similar characteristics of over-activity of one or more of the endocrine glands, such as the thyroid, pituitary, or parathyroid glands (for example). Zollinger–Ellison syndrome refers to the features due to hyperactivity and tumor production in the pancreas.

CAUSATION

Zollinger–Ellison syndrome has an autosomal dominant inheritance. The affected gene has been mapped to chromosome 11.

There is no prenatal test available. Genetic counseling, with inquiries into family members with symptoms attributable to over-activity of an endocrine gland or with tumors on such glands is advisable.

CHARACTERISTICS

Characteristics are all associated with over-secretion from the affected endocrine gland.

In Zollinger–Ellison syndrome, the pancreas is the endocrine gland involved. The pancreas is an unusual gland, as it is both an endocrine (ductless) gland and also an exocrine (ducted) gland. The ductless component secretes insulin from specialized cells—the islets of Langerhans. This process is concerned with the proper metabolism of sugars. The ducted part of the gland is involved in the breakdown of food by enzymes passed to the intestine via the pancreatic duct.

Tumors, both benign and malignant, can arise in various parts of the gland. The symptoms shown will depend on the positions of these tumors. With destruction of the insulin-producing part of the pancreas, diabetes will occur. Alternatively, excess insulin can be secreted, giving rise to attacks of hypoglycemia due to the excessive amounts of sugar being metabolized.

A specific feature of Zollinger–Ellison syndrome is excessive **acid secretion** in the stomach. This condition can give rise to peptic ulceration, which can be especially difficult to treat. Stomach pain, acid reflux, and possible bleeding from the stomach can result.

A further feature is a **raised calcium level** in the body. This fact can be useful in determining if other—nonsymptomatic—family members have the genetic susceptibility to the condition.

The biochemistry of this syndrome is complex and can be confused with other conditions of the endocrine glands.

MANAGEMENT IMPLICATIONS

Management will depend on both the site and the severity of the **tumors** involved. **Diabetes** will need to be treated, and **hypoglycemia** will require dietary changes.

For **gastric pain,** drugs, such as one of the proton pump inhibitors, will be needed to relieve the hyperacidity. In severe cases, total gastrectomy may become necessary.

THE FUTURE

The future will depend on the site and severity of the neoplasia. If the tumors are nonmalignant, the outlook is good, but, even with malignant tumors, long-term survivors of Zollinger–Ellison syndrome have been reported.

SELF-HELP GROUPS

No organization is known to be dedicated exclusively to Zollinger–Ellison syndrome. The following groups may, however, provide useful information and guidance.

National Organization for Rare Disorders (NORD)
P.O. Box 8923
New Fairfield, CT 06812-8923
800-999-6673 or 203-746-6518
http://www.nord-rdb.com/orphan
email: orphan@nord-rdb.com

National Digestive Diseases Information Clearinghouse
2 Information Way
Bethesda, MD 20892-3570
email: nddic@info.niddk.nih.gov

Glossary

Acute Sudden onset of symptoms of disease.

Adenoma sebaceum Specific rash found in tuberous sclerosis.

Amblyopia Reduced vision due to a lazy eye.

Amniocentesis Removal of amniotic fluid from around the fetus through the abdominal and uterine walls.

Amniotic fluid Fluid surrounding the fetus in the uterus.

Antibiotics Drugs used against bacterial infections.

Asymptomatic No obvious signs of a disease process.

Ataxia Loss of control of voluntary movement.

Atresia Occlusion of a normal channel in the body.

Atrial septal defects Opening between the two upper chambers of the heart.

Atrophy Wasting of any part of the body.

Audiometry Specialized test for hearing.

Autism Developmental disorder affecting communication and social skills.

Autonomic nervous system Part of the nervous system having control of routine bodily system functions.

Autosomal Concerned with bodily cells.

Avascular necrosis Death of tissue due to lack of blood supply.

Biopsy Removal of a small part of an organ for diagnostic purposes.

Bronchiectasis Lung disease following infection, often sustained in childhood.

Cataracts Clouding of the lens of the eye.

Choanal atresia Congenital blocking of one, or both, nostrils.

Chorionic villus sampling Prenatal test performed on minute parts of placental tissue.

Chromosomes Units of inheritance, of which there are normally 46 in humans.

Chronic   Long-standing disease.

Chronological age   Age from date of birth.

Cilia   Tiny hair-like structures found in many hollow organs of the body.

Coarctation   Narrowing of the aorta.

Colomba   Developmental gaps in various parts of the eye.

Conductive deafness   Specialized type of deafness not involving the nerves of hearing.

Consanguinity   Close family relationship.

Cornea   Transparent covering of the front of the eye.

Dermatologist   Medical practitioner specializing in diseases of the skin.

Developmental age   Stage of childhood development—not necessarily the same as the chronological age.

Diabetes   Disease of the pancreas resulting in dangerously high levels of blood sugar.

Dialysis   Method of removing waste products from the body in the event of kidney failure.

Dyslexia   A specific reading difficulty.

EEG   Electroencephalogram, a test measuring the electrical activity of the brain.

EKG   Electrocardiogram, a test measuring the electrical activity of the heart.

Endocarditis   Infection of the inner lining of the heart.

Enzyme   Complex organic substance causing chemical reactions in the body.

Epicanthic fold   Folds of skin from the upper eyelid over inner edge of the eye.

Epiphyseal plates   Growing parts of the bone.

Etiology   The origin, causation, and development of disease.

Eustachian tube   Tiny tube leading from the middle ear to the back of the throat.

Febrile seizures   Seizures due to a high fever in children under the age of five years.

Fistula   An abnormal connection between two organs of the body, or between an organ and the exterior.

Fontanelle   Gaps in the bones of the skull in young babies covered by fibrous tissue.

Genes   The ultimate units of inheritance found on the chromosomes.

Glaucoma   Raised pressure in the eyeball due to a fault in the drainage system.

Hernia   A weakening of muscular tissue allowing organs to protrude.

Horseshoe kidney   Congenital, U-shaped single kidney.

Hydramnios   Excess amount of amniotic fluid.

Hydrocephalus   Abnormal increase of cerebrospinal fluid in the brain.

Hydrotherapy   Special type of physical therapy undertaken in water.

Hyperactivity   Extreme activity in childhood.

Hypertension   High blood pressure.

Hypertonic   Increased muscular tone.

Hypertrophy   Excess growth of a particular tissue.

Hyperventilation   Over-breathing.

Hypocalcemia   Low blood levels of calcium.

Hypoglycemia   Low blood sugar.

Hypospadias   Abnormal opening of urethra on the penis.

Hypothyroidism   Under-function of the thyroid gland.

Hypotonic   Decreased muscular tone.

Hypsarrhythmia   Particular type of seizures.

Inguinal   Pertaining to the groin region.

Intercostal muscles   Muscles between the ribs.

Iris   Colored part of the eye.

Jaundice   Yellow coloration of the skin in liver disease.

Kyphosis   Bending of the spine in an anterior-posterior manner.

Lordosis   Normal curve of spine in region of the lower back.

Mainstream schools   Schools catering to the majority of children.
Meconium ileus   Blockage of the small intestine in the newborn.
Meiosis   Type of cell division producing sex cells.
Melanin   Substance causing skin pigmentation.
Metabolism   Chemical processes necessary to maintain life and health.
Microcephaly   A small, underdeveloped brain.
Mitosis   Type of cell division producing similar cells.
Mutations   Changes producing new effects.
Myringotomy   Surgical procedure to withdraw excess fluid from the middle ear.

Nevi   Small pigmented areas in the skin—"moles."
Nasogastric feeding   Feeding through a tube passed into the stomach via the nose.
Nystagmus   Jerky, sideways or vertical, involuntary movements of the eyes.

Ophthalmologist   Medical practitioner specializing in diseases of the eye.
Opthalmoscope   Instrument used to examine structures at the back of the eye.

Parathyroid   Endocrine glands situated at the back of the thyroid gland.
Parietal bones   One of the bones making up the skull situated at each side of the head.
Patent ductus arteriosus   Specialized type of congenital heart disease in which there is persistence of a duct between the aorta and the pulmonary artery.
Penetrance   A person inherits a specific gene, but does not necessarily develop the disorder.
Perthes disease   Childhood disease of the hip.
Phalanges   Bones of the fingers.
Photophobia   Dislike of light.

Plantar response   Reflex action of the toes when the sole of the foot is stimulated.

Platelets   Structures in the blood necessary for proper clotting.

Ptosis   Partial paralysis of the eyelids.

Pyloric stenosis   Abnormality at the lower end of the stomach.

Pyridoxine   A vitamin of the B group.

Radius   One of the bones of the forearm.

Reflexes   Involuntary responses occurring when specific parts of the body are stimulated.

Retina   Tissue at the back of the eye necessary for vision.

Scoliosis   Sideways bending of the spine.

Sensorineural deafness   Deafness due to problems with the nerves of hearing.

Sinusitis   Infection of the paranasal sinuses.

Situs invertus   Organs on the opposite side of the body to normal.

Sporadic   Condition occurring in isolated cases.

Sprengel shoulder   One shoulder higher than the other.

Systemic   Condition relating to whole bodily system or group of organs.

Talipes   Defect in the ankle—known as "clubfoot."

Testosterone   Male sex hormone.

Tetralogy of Fallot   Special type of congenital heart disease.

Thrombosis   Clotting of blood.

Thyroid   Endocrine gland situated in the front of the neck governing metabolism.

Thyroxine   Hormone secreted by the thyroid gland.

Tics   Involuntary movements of the face or body.

Trachea   Wind pipe—conducts air from the nose and mouth to the bronchi.

Tracheotomy   An artificial opening made in the trachea.

Ultrasound   Diagnostic test using ultra-high frequency sound waves to produce an image.

Urethra   Opening of the bladder to the exterior.

Venipuncture   Collection of blood from a vein.

Ventricular septal defect   Congenital abnormality in which the two lower chambers of the heart are connected.

Wilm's tumor   Specialized tumor of the kidney.

Index

abdomen, enlarged:
  in Gaucher disease, 127
  in Hurler syndrome, 157
  in Niemann–Pick disease, 217
abdominal abnormalities:
  in arthrogryposis, 39
  in Beckwith–Wiedemann syndrome, 53
  in Patau syndrome, 232
abdominal pain:
  in Fabry disease, 113
  in Gaucher disease: 128
  in nephrotic syndrome, 208
  in sickle cell anemia, 267
absent radius-thrombocytopenia. See TAR
  syndrome
achondroplasia, 9–13
acne: in Apert syndrome, 36
acoustic neuromata: in neurofibromatosis,
  214
acrocephalosyndactyly type 1. See Apert
  syndrome
acute inflammatory polyneuropathy. See
  Guillain–Barré syndrome
acute lymphatic leukemia: in Down
  syndrome, 92, 94
adnoma sebaceum: in tuberous sclerosis,
  312
adrenal gland tumors: in
  neurofibromatosis, 214
AHO. See Albright syndrome
Aicardi syndrome, 14–17
AIDS:
  and Christmas disease, 63
  and hemophilia A, 144
albinism, 18–20
Albright hereditary osteodystrophy. See
  Albright syndrome
Albright syndrome, 21–24
alcohol abuse: and fetal alcohol syndrome,
  115–17
alphagalactosidase A deficiency. See Fabry
  disease
alpha-L-iduronidase: in Hurler syndrome,
  156

Alport syndrome, 25–28
Alzheimer's disease: in Down syndrome,
  94
amblyopia. See lazy eye
AMC (arthrogryposis multiplex congenita).
  See arthrogryposis
Amsterdam dwarfism. See Cornelia de
  Lange syndrome
anal atresia:
  in Johanson–Blizzard syndrome, 167
  in VATER association, 325, 326
anemia:
  in Alport syndrome, 26
  in cystic fibrosis, 86
  in Gaucher disease, 128
  in hemolytic uremic syndrome, 139
  in Shwachman syndrome, 263
  in sickle cell anemia, 265
  in TAR syndrome, 295
  in thalassemia, 301–2
aneurysm: in Marfan syndrome, 197
Angelman syndrome, 29–31;
  compared to Prader–Willi syndrome, 240
angiokeratoma. See Fabry disease
ankylosing spondylitis, 32–34
anus, imperforate:
  in Johanson–Blizzard syndrome, 167
  in VATER association, 325, 326
Apert syndrome, 35–37;
  compared to Crouzon syndrome, 82
aphasia: in Landau–Kleffner syndrome, 179
aphasia with convulsive disorder. See
  Landau–Kleffner syndrome
apnea: in congenital central
  hypoventilation syndrome, 73
appetite, poor:
  in Alport syndrome, 26
  See also feeding problems
arachnodactyly. See Marfan syndrome
arm abnormalities:
  in Charcot–Marie–Tooth disease, 57
  in Cornelia de Lange syndrome, 77, 78
  in Ellis–van Creveld syndrome, 106
  in Goldenhar syndrome, 131